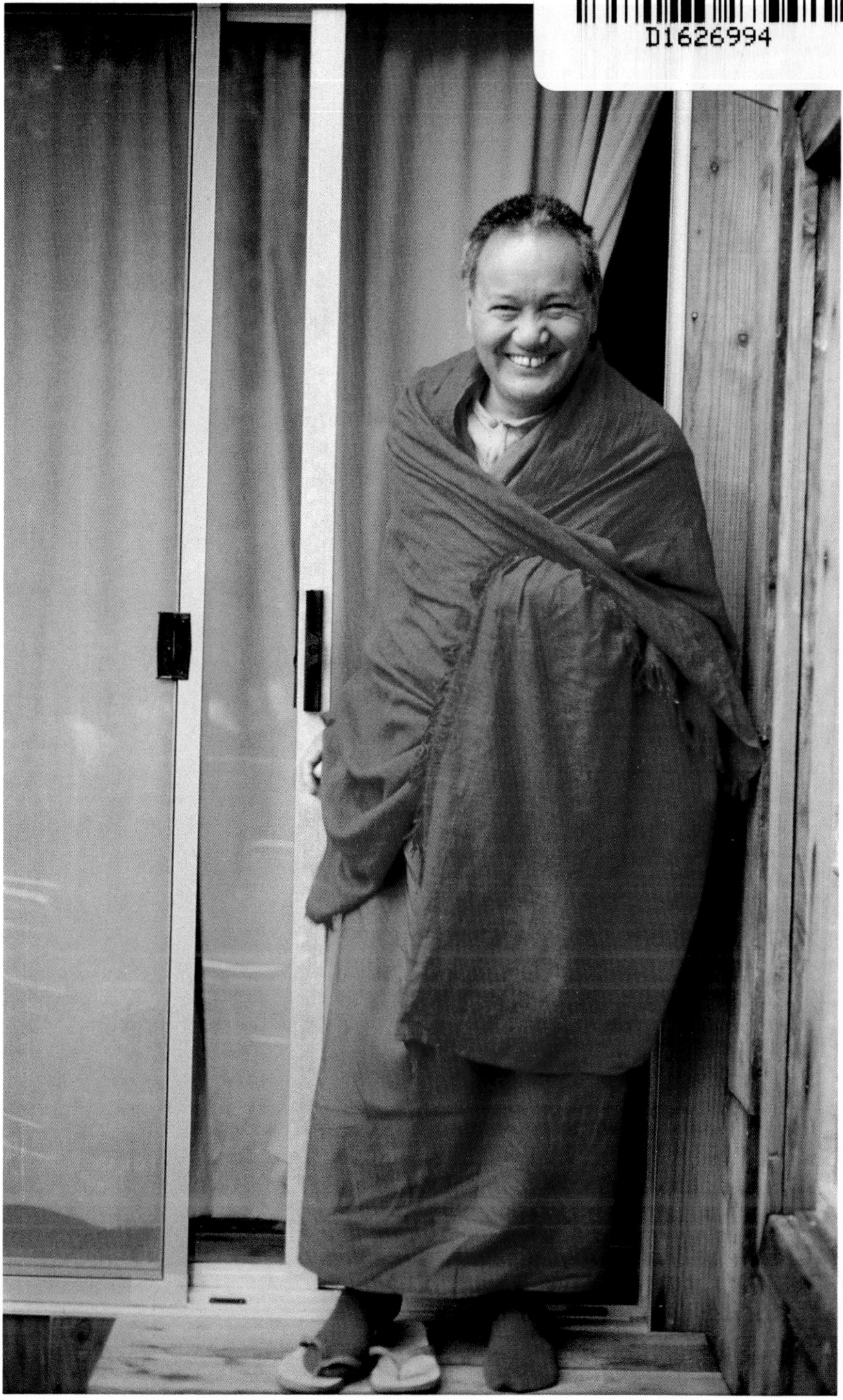

Photograph by Åge Delbanco

Lama Yeshe

The Tantric Path of Purification

THE TANTRIC PATH OF PURIFICATION

The Yoga Method of Heruka Vajrasattva

Including Complete Retreat Instructions

LAMA THUBTEN YESHE

Foreword by

LAMA THUBTEN ZOPA RINPOCHE

Compiled, edited, and annotated by Nicholas Ribush

WISDOM PUBLICATIONS • BOSTON

First published 1995
Some material previously published as Wisdom Transcripts

WISDOM PUBLICATIONS
361 NEWBURY STREET
BOSTON, MASSACHUSETTS 02115

Library of Congress Cataloging-in-Publication Data

Thubten Yeshe, 1935–1984
The tantric path of purification : the yoga method of Heruka Vajrasattva : including complete retreat instructions / Thubten Yeshe ; foreword by Thubten Zopa Rinpoche ; compiled, edited, and annotated by Nicholas Ribush.
p. cm.
Includes bibliographical references.
ISBN 0-86171-020-7 (pbk. : alk. paper) :
1. Spiritual life—Tantric Buddhism. 2. Yoga (Tantric Buddhism) 3. Heruka (Buddhist deity)—Cult. I. Ribush, Nicholas. II. Title.
BQ8938.T48 1994
294.3'443—dc20 94–30513

00 99 98 97 96
6 5 4 3 2

Cover painting: Heruka Vajrasattva *yab-yum,* by Peter Iseli
Cover photograph by Peter Studer

Set in Diacritical Garamond and Adobe Garamond Font Family

Designed by: L·J·SAWLIT

Wisdom Publications' books are printed on acid-free paper and meet the guildelines for permanence and durability of the Committee on Production Guidelines for Book Longevity of the Council on Library Resources.

Printed at Northeast Impressions, Fairfield, NJ, USA

Contents

Publisher's Acknowledgment

The publisher gratefully acknowledges the kind help of the following contributors to the Lama Yeshe Publishing Fund, whose generosity has made publication of this book possible:

Claire and Roger Ash Wheeler, Sue Bacchus, Ven. Marcel Bertels, Carl Brown, Pamela Butler, Zachary Casper, Tom Castles, Lori Cayton, Michael Childs, the Chinese Institute for Buddhist Enlightenment, Herb Cunningham, Nan Deal, Cecily Drucker, Anet Engel, Manfred Engelmann, Ian and Judy Green, Doren and Mary Harper, Pende Hawter, Norma Heavey, Ecie Hursthouse, Chrissie Jackson, John and Elaine Jackson, Jacie Keeley, Bill Kelley, Chiu Mei Lai, Ueli Minder, Jenny P'ng, Tony Page, Franco Piatti, Richard Prinz, Toby Rhodes, Beatrice Ribush, Alison and Dorian Ribush, Claire Ritter, Renee Robison, Alan Ross, Carol Royce-Wilder, Michael Schofield, John Schwartz, Sophia Su, Tom Waggoner, and anonymous friends in various places.

FOREWORD

ONE SOLUTION TO ALL OF LIFE'S PROBLEMS: THE VAJRASATTVA PURIFYING MEDITATION

I WOULD LIKE TO EXPLAIN the great importance of the Vajrasattva meditation and recitation practice. Why, it is important even for people who believe in the existence of just this life!

All life's success—including success in such ordinary things as family and friendship, business, health, wealth, and power—depends upon both purifying the negative karmic obstacles and not creating more negative karma. How do we create negative karma? When, for example, we engage in the ten negativities out of selfishness and delusion. The deluded minds are those of ignorance, attachment, and anger; the ten negativities are the three of body—killing, stealing, and sexual misconduct—the four of speech—lying, slandering, hurting others, and gossiping—and the three of mind—covetousness, ill-will, and wrong views. According to the natural law of karma, if you hurt others, you hurt yourself.

It works the other way, too. If you want others to love you, you must first love others. If you help or benefit others, naturally they will help or benefit you. The cause and effect of karma is as simple as this. In terms of the Vajrasattva purification practice, which is more powerful than negative karma, it can prevent you from experiencing the problems that the negative karma would otherwise have brought. Thus the practice of purification is one of the most important solutions to problems, and is extremely necessary, even for people who believe there is just one life.

Unfortunately, such people's hearts are usually not open to learning new things about the reality of life or the nature of phenomena—new philosophies, new subjects. They won't even analyze new possibilities. All this serves only to prevent them from experiencing either temporal or ultimate happiness. If you don't want relationship problems, business failures, illnesses such as cancer or AIDS, notoriety, or the criticism of others, the practice of Vajrasattva is extremely important.

When it comes to spiritual growth, the Vajrasattva purification practice becomes far more important. For example, as Manjushri advised Lama Tsong Khapa, "The way to actualize the path to enlightenment quickly is to do three things: practice purification and the accumulation of merit, make single-pointed requests to the guru, and train the mind in the path to enlightenment."

For these reasons, the practice of Vajrasattva is very common in all four traditions of Tibetan Buddhism—Nyingma, Kagyu, Sakya, and Geluk—where it is used to purify obstacles, obscurations, negative karma, and illness. The root tantra *Dorje Gyän* (*Vajra Ornament*) states that if you are always unconscious and careless, even small negativities cause great damage to your body, speech, and mind, just as the venom of a poisonous snake will spread rapidly throughout your body, getting worse and worse every day, endangering your life.

The great enlightened being Pabongka Dechen Nyingpo said that if you have killed even a tiny insect and not purified that negativity by the end of the day by a practice such as the Vajrasattva purification, the weight of that karma will have doubled by the next day. On the third day it will have doubled again, and by fifteen days will have become as heavy as the karma of killing a human being. By eighteen days it will have increased 131,072 times. So you can see, as the weeks and months and years go by, one tiny little negative karma will have multiplied over and over again until sooner or later it has become like a mountain the size of this earth. By the time of death, it will have become so very heavy.

Here, of course, I am talking about just one small negative karma, but every day we accumulate many, many negative karmas of body, speech, and mind. The weight of each tiny negative karma created each day multiplies over and over again, making it unimaginably heavy. And there's no question that every day, besides those small negative karmas, we also create many gross negativities. Thus we have accumulated many heavy negative karmas in this life, and in all our beginningless previous lives as well. If you contemplate the continuous multiplication of all these karmas it is unimaginably unimaginable!

The *Dorje Gyän* also states that if you recite the one hundred syllable Vajrasattva mantra twenty-one times every day, negative karmas are prevented from multiplying. The great, sublime realized beings also explain that this is the way to purify whatever downfalls and transgressions you have accumulated. Furthermore, His Holiness Trijang Rinpoche, who is actually Heruka himself, has explained that if recited twenty-eight times each day, the short Vajrasattva mantra (OM VAJRASATTVA HUM) has incredible purifying power. It not only has the power to prevent any negative karma created that day from multiplying, but it can also completely purify all negativities you have ever created—in that day, in that life, and even since your beginningless rebirths.

So these are some of the incredible advantages, or benefits, of practicing the Vajrasattva recitation and meditation. Moreover, it is taught that if you recite the long Vajrasattva mantra one hundred thousand times you can purify even broken root vows of highest yoga tantra. Thus there's no question that you can purify broken root *pratimoksha* (individual liberation) and bodhisattva vows through this technique.

Experienced meditators have advised that, in general, it is more important to put your everyday life's effort into the practice of purification—this is the way to attain spiritual realizations. The Kadampa geshe Dolbowa said that if you practice purification and accumulation of merit continuously and turn your mind to the path, *lam-rim* realizations that you thought would take one hundred years to achieve will come to you in just seven. Such are the inspiring instructions of the highly experienced meditators who attained the various levels of the path to enlightenment.

Lama Atisha used to say that there are an inconceivable number of doors to downfall for tantric practitioners who have taken highest yoga tantra initiations. For example, simply looking at an ordinary object such as a vase and seeing it as ordinary is a downfall. Just as a clean mandala left on the altar quickly gets covered in dust, so does your mental continuum collect piles of negativities in a very short time. However, don't conclude from hearing this that taking secret mantra initiations must make it impossible to reach enlightenment. Lama Atisha said that it is only people who don't know that secret mantra contains incredibly skillful means of purifying downfalls who think that way.

He said, "Just as one stone can scatter one hundred birds, there is the special skillful means called the practice of Vajrasattva." What Lama Atisha was saying was that on the one hand, in just one minute, it is so easy to accumulate a torrential downpour of downfalls and negativities—for example, looking at an object as ordinary—but on the other, there is the skillful means of tantra, the practice of Vajrasattva. This one practice will purify the countless negativities of broken root and branch vows, and in this way you can develop your mind in the path to enlightenment.

Therefore, the practice of Vajrasattva is extremely important—both for those who accept the existence of reincarnation and karma and for those who do not.

The Vajrasattva commentary in this book is an experiential instruction given by my guru, Lama Yeshe, who even to the ordinary view was a great yogi, and who took care of me like a father takes care of his only child. He gave me not only the means of living, such as food and clothing, but also guided me in the Dharma for more than thirty years.

Whoever studies this book and gets inspired to do the Vajrasattva practice and retreat is also being guided by Lama's compassion: he is liberating you from many eons of negative karma, many inconceivable eons of suffering in the lower realms, and the human and deva realms as well, and leading you to liberation and full enlightenment.

May whoever sees, touches, remembers, or even thinks or talks about this book never be born in the lower realms, receive only perfect human rebirths, meet a perfectly qualified Mahayana virtuous friend, practice the Vajrasattva purification every day, and quickly achieve Guru Vajrasattva's enlightened state. This is my wish.

Thank you very much.

Thubten Zopa

Preface

LAMA THUBTEN YESHE (1935–1984) first gave the Heruka Vajrasattva initiation and practice to about twenty-five of his Western students at Kopan Monastery, Nepal, in April 1974.

Details of Lama Yeshe's remarkable life can now be found in several places, from Vicki Mackenzie's excellent book, *Reincarnation: The Boy Lama,* and the second Wisdom Magazine, to the Introductions, Prefaces, and Afterwords of his previously published works: *Wisdom Energy* and *Introduction to Tantra.* Adèle Hulse is writing an official biography for publication by Wisdom.

But perhaps the most eloquent accounts of Lama Yeshe's extraordinary qualities are those given by Lama Thubten Zopa Rinpoche, Lama Yeshe's chief and heart disciple, in the Wisdom Transcript *The Kindness of the Guru,* and in his tributes to Lama Yeshe after Lama passed away in 1984.[1]

Not only was Lama Yeshe the quintessential *vajra* master, but he was also the inspiration behind the creation of the Foundation for the Preservation of the Mahayana Tradition (FPMT), a worldwide organization of Buddhist meditation and teaching centers, both urban and rural, monasteries, retreat facilities, healing centers, and publishing houses.

I first met Lama in November 1972 while attending the third Kopan meditation course, my first. The teachings were being given by Lama Zopa Rinpoche, and most of the fifty students in attendance were unaware that there was another lama at Kopan. Someone found out that I was a physician, and about a week into the course, I was asked to go see "Lama," who had an infection on his leg. I was taken round the back of the old house at Kopan (now, sadly, demolished), where a humble Tibetan monk, smiling broadly, greeted me with profuse thanks for nothing I'd yet done. But he knew what I didn't—that my life had already begun to change completely.

When my first shot of penicillin squirted all over the room instead of into Lama's buttock, I was invited, with a smile, to return to "try again tomorrow, dear." Thus I saw Lama daily for the next week or so, my Dharma career beginning to flourish even as my medical one began to peter out. Eighteen months later, the now-famous Kopan courses—held twice a year, back then—were attracting well over two hundred people at a time, most of them young Westerners traveling in India and Nepal. Twenty of us, inspired by the peerless example of our teachers, had taken ordination as monks and nuns. In the spring of 1974, just after the sixth Kopan course and several years of *sutra* teachings on the graduated path to enlightenment, Lama felt we were ready for *tantra.* He chose the purification practice of Heruka Vajrasattva, and compiled for our use a *sadhana,* or method of accomplishment, from the Chakrasamvara tantra. He then gave a five-lecture commentary on the sadhana and an extensive discourse on how to make a meditational retreat.

This book comprises Lama's commentary on the Vajrasattva practice (see below), detailed retreat instructions based mainly on that initial teaching, six occasional discourses, mostly given as introductions to Heruka Vajrasattva initiations at FPMT centers around the world, and two commentaries on the *Heruka Vajrasattva Tsok* that Lama himself composed in 1982. In the Appendices will be found the sadhana and tsok text in Tibetan script, phoneticized Tibetan, for ease of chanting, and English, and a method for blessing the offering to the local spirits, the *shi-dak torma.* But it must be emphasized, as Lama says in his introduction, to do the Heruka Vajrasattva practice you require a highest yoga tantra initiation and instruction from a fully qualified lama.

In this vein, readers should also note that since the teachings in this book are from the oral tradition and aimed at practitioners, Sanskrit and Tibetan terms have not been rendered with scholars in mind but in phonetics approximating their correct pronunciation, devoid of diacritics.

Another point to make is that in these teachings, Lama Yeshe frequently uses the word "Westerners," which reflects his audience at the time and has not been edited out. However, non-Western readers should not feel left out, as Lama's wisdom and compassion radiated in the ten directions with complete impartiality.

Lama's 1974 commentary was taped and transcribed by the monks and nuns of the International Mahayana Institute, prior to their undertaking the Heruka Vajrasattva retreat in the summer of 1974. I spent more than four months with this commentary in the Charok Cave at Lawudo, not far from the Lawudo Gompa, the site of the hermitage of the Lawudo Lama, of whom Lama Zopa Rinpoche is the reincarnation. This was the high point of my life, and I would recommend making retreat with Lama's commentary to anybody. And having ten or so vajra brothers and sisters up and down the Lawudo mountain around me, doing the same practice, was a great inspiration. It was a wonderful time.

Simultaneously, twenty or so meditators inaugurated group retreat within the FPMT at Kopan Gompa, and three-month Heruka Vajrasattva group retreats are still conducted annually at Tushita Retreat Center, above Dharamsala, India, and Milarepa Center, Vermont, USA, and occasionally at other centers.

After the retreat, Lama worked with Ven. Marcel Bertels and Ven. Yeshe Khadro to augment both the initial sadhana and commentary. For almost twenty years, scores of Heruka Vajrasattva retreaters have relied upon Marcel's excellent edition of the commentary, which has been reprinted in transcript form many times by both Kopan Monastery and Wisdom. It forms the basis of Parts 1 and 2 of this book.

I began work on *The Tantric Path of Purification* after Lama Yeshe had appointed me Wisdom's editorial director in 1981. Following Lama's teachings on the Six Yogas of Naropa at Istituto Lama Tzong Khapa in early 1983, seven of us, as detailed by Jon Landaw in *Introduction to Tantra,* got together at an editing retreat near Cecina, Italy, to work on a number of Lama's other teachings for publication. Among many other things, we learned that so unique was Lama's "extremely creative use of English," as retreater Robin Brentano tactfully put it, that editing his words was akin to translation. The challenge presented by editing Lama's teachings is to come up with a text that is true to his meaning, is grammatically correct, and sounds like Lama. Those of us presented with this challenge do the best we can!

I read my first draft of the main commentary to Lama at Tushita Retreat Center in April 1983, and he made many corrections, additions, and suggestions. I treasure my tapes of those meetings, as I do my memories of all the other times I spent with Lama. All his suggestions have been incorporated in this book.

I edited the later teachings—Lama's occasional Heruka Vajrasattva lectures and his commentaries to the Heruka Vajrasattva Tsok offering he composed—in 1993, at Kinglake, Victoria, Australia.

Lama Yeshe was a great advocate of the Heruka Vajrasattva purification practice. He once expressed the hope that all his students would make the time to do the retreat at least once before they died. After Lama passed away, according to his wishes, a group of students maintained a round-the-clock schedule of Heruka Vajrasattva practice for twelve months at Kopan Monastery, and for shorter periods at Ösel Ling Retreat Center, Spai, and Mahamudra Center, New Zealand.

Out of Lama's great compassion and his students' somewhat shaky karma, on February 12, 1985 he returned to earth as Lama Tenzin Ösel Rinpoche, and we pray for the day that he will once again teach the Heruka Vajrasattva practice to his disciples and, perhaps, correct whatever errors have been introduced into this book.

ACKNOWLEDGMENTS

"Thank you, Rinpoche, for changing my life," I said to Lama Zopa Rinpoche at the end of my first Kopan meditation course (he just laughed). All of us in the FPMT give continual thanks to Lama Zopa Rinpoche, our shining beacon of wisdom and compassion and a living example of enlightened realizations. When Lama Yeshe passed away, Rinpoche seamlessly maintained the development of the FPMT until it now comprises more than seventy centers in seventeen countries around the world, while continuing to lead an ever-growing number of international disciples spiritually, both by his incomparable demeanor and by his profound teachings.

This project and many others have benefited and will benefit even more in the future from the exceptional work done by Peter and Nicole Kedge and Ven. Ailsa Cameron in establishing and maintaining the Wisdom Archive of teachings by Lama Thubten Yeshe and Lama Thubten Zopa Rinpoche. This computerized diamond mine will continue to produce teachings for the benefit of all sentient beings for a long time to come, and as the publisher of those teachings, we are extremely grateful for their dedicated work.

Without listing what they did to help, but they did plenty, I would also like to thank Ven. Geshe Lama Lhundrub Rigsel, director of Kopan Monastery, Ven. Marcel Bertels, Ven. Yeshe Khadro, Martin Willson, Ven. Connie Miller, T. Yeshe, Ven. Sangye Khadro, Ven. Thubten Pemo, Ven. Thubten Wongmo, Ursula Bernis, Ven. Ann McNeil, Ven. Max Mathews, Jonathan Landaw, Ven. Robina Courtin, Ven. Roger Kunsang, Tim McNeill, Thubten Chödak, Piero Cerri, members of the Cecina Mare editing retreat, Mary Moffat, Cookie Claire Ritter, my mother Beatrice Ribush, Dorian and Alison Ribush, Wendy Cook, Ven. Geshe Tsulga (Tsultrim Chöpel), David Molk, Ven. George Churinoff, and Vincent Montenegro. Thanks are also due to the FPMT centers where the teachings in this book were given, and to the dedicated students who transcribed the tapes. We are especially grateful to Peter Iseli for the beautiful painting of Heruka Vajrasattva that adorns the cover of this book, which in turn was beautifully designed by Lisa Sawlit.

Nicholas Ribush

Editor's Introduction

Purification, the Four Opponent Powers, and the Practice of Vajrasattva

Before Lama Yeshe began giving tantric initiations and teachings, as mentioned above, he made sure his Western students were well versed in the three principal aspects of the sutra path—renunciation, *bodhicitta,* and the right view of emptiness (*sunyata*)—by having his main disciple, Lama Thubten Zopa Rinpoche, teach intensive, one-month retreats on the lam-rim (graduated path to enlightenment) twice a year. After six of these "Kopan courses," Lama decided that his students were ready for highest (*maha-anuttara*) yoga tantra and agreed to initiate them into the purification practice of Heruka Vajrasattva.

In his *Introduction to Tantra* and *The Bliss of Inner Fire,* Lama Yeshe has explained the relationship between sutra and tantra, the two main divisions of Mahayana Buddhism. Further information may be found in the pages of this book and in the titles listed under Suggested Further Reading. However, to place purification in context, we need only recall Manjushri's advice to Lama Je Tsong Khapa: to attain spiritual realizations one must combine meditation on the path to enlightenment with purification, accumulation of merit, and praying to one's guru as a buddha. As Lama explains, the yoga method of Heruka Vajrasattva involves all of these, with special emphasis upon the aspect of purification.

Without purifying your mind to prepare it for spiritual realizations, you will make little progress toward enlightenment. The purification methods revealed in this book are among the most powerful ever taught. In Buddhist practice, purification is a science based upon an understanding of the psycho-mechanics of karma, or action, the law of cause and effect, and entails the application of the four opponent powers.[2] Sometimes called "confession," purification is very different from what Christians will understand by the term, although some parallels may be found.

Actions of body, speech, and mind leave imprints upon the consciousness, like seeds planted in a field. When the conditions are right, these imprints ripen into experiences. Positive imprints, or good karma, bring the result of happiness; negative imprints, or bad karma, bring suffering. The difference between the two is very clearly explained in Lama Zopa Rinpoche's book, *The Door to Satisfaction.*

Every action has four aspects that determine whether it is complete or incomplete: motivation, object, performance, and completion. For example, to be complete, the action of killing would require the motivation, or intention, to kill; a sentient being as the object to be killed; performance of the action, either directly or indirectly, that is, doing it oneself or ordering someone else to do it; and completion of the action, with the other sentient being dying before the killer.

If an action is complete in all four aspects, it becomes what is called a throwing karma, an action that can determine your state of rebirth by throwing you into one of the six samsaric realms. If one or more of the four branches is missing, the action becomes a completing karma, determining the quality of the experiences you will have in this and future lives. A completing karma brings three types of result: the result similar to the cause in experience, the result similar to the cause in habit, and the environmental results. Thus, a complete negative karma has four suffering results. For example, the four results of killing could be, respectively, rebirth in a hell, a short life plagued with illness, a tendency to kill other beings, and rebirth in a very dangerous place.

Although all this applies equally to positive as well as negative actions, we are focusing here on the latter in the context of purification. The four opponent powers work—and are all necessary— because each one counters one of the four negative karmic results. The first power—taking refuge and generating bodhicitta—is called the power of the object, or the power of dependence, and purifies the throwing karma that causes us to be reborn in the three lower realms. It is called the power of dependence because our recovery depends upon the object that hurt us. For example, to get up after you have fallen over and hurt yourself, you depend upon the same ground that hurt you. Similarly, almost all the negative karma we create has as its objects either holy objects or sentient beings. In order to purify it we take refuge in holy objects and generate bodhicitta for the sake of all sentient beings.

The second power is the power of release, which counteracts the result similar to the cause in experience. The third power is the power of the remedy, which is the antidote to the environmental result. Finally, the fourth power is that of indestructible determination, by which we overcome our lifetime-to-lifetime tendency to habitually create negativities again and again. Thus, in neutralizing the four different results of negative karma, the four opponent powers purify them completely, preventing us from ever having to experience their suffering results. This kind of explicit logic lies behind all Buddhist practice and explains, in part, why Buddhism is so appealing to the intelligent, well-educated spiritual seeker of today.

The third power embraces many different kinds of remedy, from making prostrations to building stupas to reciting the one hundred syllable Vajrasattva mantra to meditating on emptiness. Ideally, several of these are practiced simultaneously. In the commentary, Lama Yeshe emphasizes realization of emptiness as the ultimate purification and shows how correct practice of the sadhana, which contains the four opponent powers, organically leads up to the actual remedy in this practice, recitation of the mantra. His detailed explanation of the Mahayana technique of inner refuge as part of the power of the object is both exceptional and unique.

As Lama Yeshe makes abundantly clear, the most effective—although not the only—way to practice the Vajrasattva purification method is in retreat. Therefore, he has given detailed instructions on every aspect of group and individual retreat, instructions that will, in fact, be useful for those making any kind of retreat.

The six discourses in part 3 are wonderful, bite-sized Dharma discourses that Vajrasattva retreaters will find especially useful to read during session breaks. However, none of us reading these excellent talks will fail to be inspired by Lama's uniquely motivating energy.

Finally, all practitioners of mother tantra are required to offer tsok on the tenth and twenty-fifth days of the Tibetan month, and most do so by practicing the *Guru Puja.* However, the *Heruka Vajrasattva Tsok* that Lama composed is a also perfect means of fulfilling that commitment, especially when in Vajrasattva retreat, and it was Lama's hope that his students and others would include this tsok puja as part of their regular practice.

It is often said that the lam-rim teachings are like a meal ready to eat—that the logical the way in which they are arranged makes it easy to see the entire Dharma path and to know in which order the vast array of Buddhist meditations should be undertaken in order for the practitioner to reach enlightenment. In *The Tantric Path of Purification,* Lama Yeshe has prepared a tantric banquet for all to enjoy.

Introduction

Intellectuals, Beware!

During an initiation, the guru calls upon the divine energy of the universe, which manifests as divine, blissful wisdom in the shape of the particular deity—in this case, Heruka Vajrasattva. This energy activates a force largely dormant in the disciple's nervous system, which now awakens and begins to vibrate. If you generate the proper altruistic state of mind and an understanding of emptiness, and recite the Vajrasattva mantra, you maintain and augment the vibration activated by the guru. If then, through a period of silent contemplation, you induce a calm, reflective mind, free of your usual flow of obscuring, uncontrolled thoughts, your inner wisdom will automatically reveal itself.

But, a word of caution to the intellectual. Reading tantric teachings on your own, without the power of the appropriate initiation, is just an intellectual pastime—only by practicing correctly, under the guidance of a fully qualified and experienced teacher, can you evolve beyond the intellect, beyond conceptual thought, into the true wisdom of a pure, spontaneous being. I am not trying to be mysterious or exclusive here but simply saying that if you think that you can understand, let alone experience, the methods of tantric yoga merely by reading books, you are deceiving yourself—like a terminally ill person doctoring himself with the same methods that made him ill in the first place.

The yoga method of Heruka Vajrasattva should be practiced only by those who have received the initiation and oral commentary from a properly qualified vajra master. Although the commentary published here is potentially of limitless value and should be studied thoroughly before you practice the methods it describes, you must take the initiation and receive some instruction from your guru. Otherwise, instead of giving you the direct experience you seek, it will become a dry, intellectual exercise of relatively little benefit.

The great Tibetan yogi Dharmavajra explained that the highest (maha-anuttara) yoga tantra initiation of Heruka Vajrasattva is a special feature of the Gelug tradition of Tibetan Buddhism. Highest yoga tantra contains methods by which you can reach enlightenment in a single lifetime or even, as in Lama Tsong Khapa's case, three short years. Of course, these profound teachings have never been published, but the methods still exist, undegenerated, in the minds of certain practitioners. These esoteric teachings of Lord Buddha can be transmitted only through unobstructed inner communication between vajra guru and disciple. Few people realize that such powerful methods can still be found in the teachings of the Geluk school.

A whole tradition of Tibetan yogis has made the yoga method of Heruka Vajrasattva a living experience. Before you can actualize the generation (*kye-rim*) and completion (*dzok-rim*) stages of highest yoga tantra, you must purify yourself: practicing Heruka Vajrasattva is one of the most powerful ways of doing so. After taking the initiation, you enter retreat, in which you recite one hundred thousand Vajrasattva (one hundred syllable) mantras. This allows you to practice the two stages of tantra more effectively. If you have not purified the old defiled habits of your body, speech, and mind, even if you put enormous effort into meditating on the path to enlightenment, you will not gain realizations because there are too many obstacles in your way.

Therefore, you should alternate purification with lam-rim meditation. Even trying to achieve single-pointed concentration (*vipasyana*) without purification causes you to become frustrated and feel hopeless and discouraged with your lack of progress. This is because you have not recognized or dealt with the obstacles thrown up by your habitual wrong-conception mind and its by-products—defiled body and speech.

Some misguided practitioners try to experience emptiness simply by rejecting the existence of all phenomena, obsessed with the idea that sunyata is some kind of vague nothingness. If you want to actualize the right view of emptiness in accordance with, for example, the Madhyamaka or Zen schools of Buddhist philosophy, you have to practice both method and wisdom. Many people have great interest in wisdom but none at all in method. They are like a bird trying to fly with a broken wing.

Whenever you encounter interruptions and obstacles to your practice, don't get discouraged or depressed. Realize instead that you need to purify, and for a time, concentrate more on method than wisdom. In due course you will gain the realizations that you seek.

Part 1

THE MAIN COMMENTARY

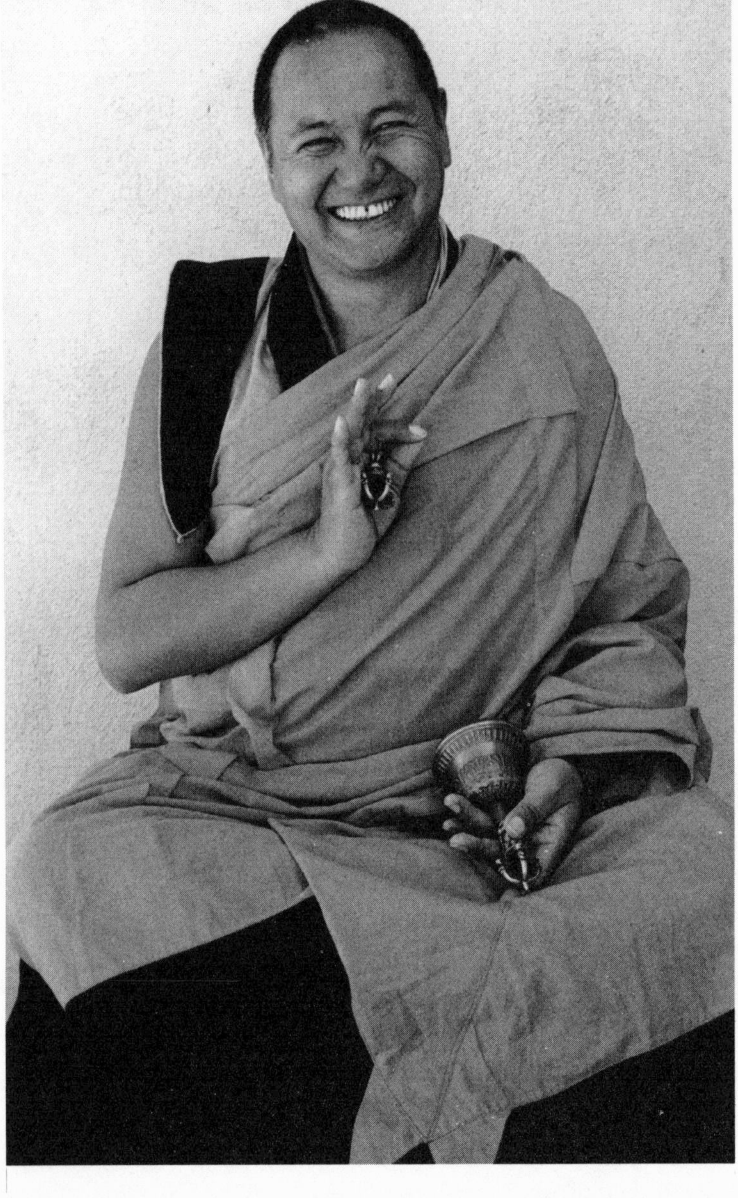

Photograph by Carol Royce-Wilder

1

Why and How We Purify

This teaching has come at your request, not from my saying, "I want to give you teachings; come here and listen!" In your studies on the graduated path to enlightenment you have come to understand how powerful your minds are and how they create powerful positive and negative actions. Aware of this, you have examined your lives and seen the nature of the actions of your body, speech, and mind. Thus, with knowledge-wisdom, you have requested this teaching to be able to purify the negative forces within you.

The way you have requested this teaching is also very good. Based on your understanding of the characteristics of the negative mind, your request is neither ignorant nor emotional. Since you are fortunate, intelligent, and wise enough to be able to practice this powerful yoga,method and thereby destroy your negative energy forces completely, I feel that giving you this teaching will be of great benefit.

First of all, you are very fortunate even to see that there really *is* a solution to the negative actions that arise from the ignorant mind. Consider how most people are unaware of how they create actions; nor do they understand the difference between positive and negative actions and their results of happiness and suffering. You know all this—that's why you are very lucky. Even when people discover this evolution, it is very difficult for them to see how to purify and free themselves completely from the cycle of cause and effect to which they are bound. This is not easy; it takes a long time. You really are fortunate to have come to the conclusion that you can purify yourselves.

Furthermore, you are very lucky that your wisdom can grasp the profound methods of tantric yoga. This, too, is very difficult. How difficult is it? Well, when Westerners first meet the Dharma they cannot even understand the purpose of making prostrations: "Why should I do prostrations? Sorry, that's not for me." Prostrations are so simple, so easy to understand! The profound methods of tantric yoga are extremely deep. It is highly worthwhile for you to do these powerful purification practices.

Let me put this another way. We often find that when we meditate on the lam-rim—the path to liberation and enlightened realizations—we encounter many hindrances. We cannot understand why it is so difficult to meditate, to control our minds, to gain realizations. "Why do I meet with so many obstacles whenever I try to do something positive? Leading a worldly life was much easier than this. Even an hour's meditation is so difficult." Many such thoughts and questions arise.

It is not just a lack of wisdom. It is that over countless lives the negative energy forces of our body, speech, and mind have accumulated such that now they fill us like a vast ocean. If they were to manifest in physical form, they would occupy all of space. By contrast, our small intellectual knowledge-wisdom is as weak as the light of a flickering little candle. A little candle isn't much help on a dark and windy night.

Our tiny candle-like knowledge-wisdom cannot control or release us from the overwhelming force of our negative mind. Thus, it is the energy of our wrong conceptions, our negative mind, that makes it difficult for us to actualize the everlasting peaceful path of liberation and to receive realizations. Therefore, we need a powerful purification practice like the tantric yoga method of Heruka Vajrasattva to destroy both the energy forces of the ignorant mind and the negative actions of body and speech that arise from it.

The yoga method of Heruka Vajrasattva has the power to purify all negative energy, which is the main thing preventing you from actualizing the path. This impure energy creates both physical and mental hindrances, and also leaves certain imprints. Philosophically, we say that these are neither mind nor form. If you are interested in this, you can investigate at another time what kind of phenomenon they are. The reason I bring it up is that when I'm talking about negativity here my meaning might be different from your previous understanding of the term. Most Westerners think that negativity refers to just the gross level of the emotions. It goes much deeper than that.

Take, for example, the physical body. The first time people come to a meditation course they have great trouble in just sitting. Something in their nervous system pulls their energy down to the base of their spine. The reason we recommend the classical cross-legged meditation posture is that when you sit with your back straight, the psychic energy flows properly, and thus, it is much easier for you to control your mind. However, this change in your nervous system makes it feel as if all your energy is falling down from your crown chakra to your lower chakra. This makes some people terrified that they are losing their minds. Not only do new students have trouble sitting, they also have to concentrate their minds for long periods listening to totally new ideas, which can also be very unsettling. These physical and mental problems really make them wonder why on earth they are sitting there.

The pressure in the lower chakra is caused by negative physical energy, which comes from the negative mind. In Mahayana Buddhism we place less emphasis on such physical reactions and focus on the root of all problems, the ignorant, negative mind.

While insight meditation on the graduated path is the actual way to liberation, when you feel that you cannot meditate—there are too many interruptions, you cannot do anything, you cannot solve your problems—remember that there is something else you can do to remove obstacles to your progress: purification. In the experience of Tibetan lamas, sessions of insight meditation on the path should alternate with sessions of a powerful purification practice, such as the yoga method of Heruka Vajrasattva. This combined approach ensures that you will gain the realizations you seek without frustration.

But do not have unrealistic expectations: "Today I'm completely negative, tonight I meditate, tomorrow I'll be completely pure." You cannot purify yourself overnight. Not only are such expectations wrong, they themselves become obstacles. Especially when retreating you should not expect anything—just relax. All you need to feel is that in this life you will act as positively as possible. If you can do that, good results will come whether you expect them or not. You won't have to keep asking your lama for a prediction: "If I control my body, speech, and mind, avoid all negativities, and do only good, will I experience positive results?" Many students do this. Why? Because they don't understand karma. If you always act wisely and keep your actions positive, what need is there to ask?

Just think: "From now until I die, whether realizations come to me or not, I shall act as positively as I can, trying to make my life as beneficial as possible for myself and others." What more can you expect? That sort of expectation is far more reasonable and logical than thinking, "If I meditate for a month I'll become Heruka Vajrasattva." Such expectations only disturb your mind.

Even though you might have created negative actions all your life, a positive mind at the time of death guarantees that you will not be reborn in the lower realms. You receive this internal guarantee when you purify your negativities. It is not like ordinary guarantees; you can trust it completely. In the world, things are constantly changing. You can never trust worldly, paper guarantees. But the internal guarantee of positive karma ensures that at the time of death you will be able to control your mind and not fall under the influence of negative minds such as desire and hatred.

In order to gain higher realizations, it is most important to practice the powerful methods of purification found in the Vajrayana path. Many lamas have found that purification overcomes the hindrances of both negative energy and its imprints.

While other Vajrasattva practices emphasize physical purification, the Heruka Vajrasattva yoga method is set up to emphasize mental purification. This makes it especially powerful.

THE FOUR OPPONENT POWERS

The Heruka Vajrasattva sadhana is divided into three parts: taking refuge, generating bodhicitta, and the actual yoga method. Why are taking refuge and generating bodhicitta parts of this purification practice? Because negative actions are usually created in relation either to holy objects such as the Three Jewels of refuge, or to other sentient beings.

You can see for yourself how this is true. Just check. Most of your problems arise from the people around you, not from bricks, rocks, or trees. And the most common problems can be found between people who are close to each other—the closer the connection the more the mental complications. For example, if you keep away from tar, you'll be okay; but if you touch it, it will get all over you, will be hard to get rid of, and will cause you much difficulty. In the same way, proximity to other people can lead to sticky situations.

Some simple examples of common negativities will clarify this. We ourselves, the subject of the action, act under the influence of our negative minds, but we usually need an object upon which to act. For example, when we kill, there has to be another being whose life we take; when we steal, there has to be an owner of the thing we take; when we lie, there has to be someone to lie to. Of course, our ignorant, dissatisfied, greedy, selfish mind is always there, but other beings have to be there, too. In this way we create negativities in dependence upon others. We purify such negative karma by generating bodhicitta.

We also create negativities in dependence upon holy objects. Sometimes, with negative mind, we might criticize a buddha, denigrate a bodhisattva, treat books or statues incorrectly, or complain about monks or nuns. There are countless ways to create such negative karma, and we purify it by taking refuge in Buddha, Dharma, and Sangha .

To generate bodhicitta we must feel unbearable great compassion for all sentient beings, irrespective of their species, race, nationality, or philosophical or religious beliefs. As well, we must have the strong, enthusiastic will to lead them to perfect enlightenment, taking the responsibility for doing so upon ourselves alone. Just having this attitude releases us from much negativity.

For example, you have a very strong but uncontrolled karmic connection with your parents. Although they have been most kind to you, you cause them great suffering. You cannot cut the connection with your parents simply by saying that you are completely fed up with them and never want to see them again and running off to the mountains. It is not enough to separate yourself from them physically. To finish the karma with your parents you have to purify it by having great compassion for them and generating bodhicitta with them in mind. Similarly, you can't cut your karmic connection with other people intellectually, by just saying you're finished with them and never want to see them again. These links have to be severed by purification.

The best way to purify negativities is by using the four opponent powers. The first of these is the *power of the object,* which means taking refuge and generating bodhicitta. In the practice I am describing here, the object of refuge is Heruka Vajrasattva, who is oneness with the Three Jewels of refuge: Buddha, Dharma, and Sangha . We can also say he is oneness with the guru, the absolute guru, but I'll talk more about that later. His divine wisdom understands the nature of both positive and negative energy forces. He becomes your liberator, and you go to him for refuge.

The second power is the *power of release.* It is sometimes called the power of regret, but this may have a misleading connotation. This power derives from wisdom and is not some kind of emotional sorrow or guilt, which are feelings that merely perpetuate our problems since they cause us to accumulate more negative propensities. Think of a person who suddenly realizes that he has just swallowed poison: he wants to take the antidote right away. The power of release is the wisdom that understands the negative repercussions of unwholesome actions so well that the moment you become aware that you have created a negative action, you want to purify it immediately.

The third is the *power of remedy.* It is with this power that you actually counteract the force of your amassed negativities. With single-pointed concentration on Heruka Vajrasattva—the manifestation of blissful, transcendental, divine wisdom who is oneness with your guru—you do the yoga method and powerfully recite the purifying mantra. This practice is the remedy.

I'm not sure that the fourth power can be succinctly translated into English. It is something like the *power of indestructible determination,* where you have great determination never, never, never again to be influenced by your defiled habits. It is not so much a vow or a promise or a resolution or a decision. Simultaneous with the power of the remedy you have this great determination never to create any negative actions again. There is something complete about it. It is firm and strong and comes from wisdom. Within you there is a subtle energy that protects you from moral falls. It is far more than an intellectually motivated decision: it is a force that totally counteracts the old habits, a realization that instinctively protects you. Of course, this power has degrees, but when fully developed it offers perfect protection.

For example, when you take the eight Mahayana precepts for a day, at the time of the ordination in the early morning you generate the great determination to keep the vows intact. From that moment on you must practice perfect awareness and maintain it throughout the day. Determination to keep the precepts at the time of the ceremony alone is not enough; it has to be maintained minute by minute for the duration of the commitment. Otherwise, as soon as the ordination ceremony is over, you will fall straight back into your old samsaric ways, almost unconscious, completely unaware of what you are doing.

Vows are not broken by instantaneous mental actions. The motivation for an action that will break a vow evolves gradually in the mind. You have a long history of similar uncontrolled energy patterns. Therefore, if your early morning determination is accompanied by exceptional continuous conscious awareness, there is no way you can break your vows. Within you there is that very subtle, accumulated energy that completely protects you from defiled actions.

KARMA

The same thing applies to following the law of karma. When we take refuge, our main obligation is to keep our karma straight, to avoid defiled, negative actions. But often we cannot do so, even though we understand on an intellectual level that if we keep on creating such actions again and again, we shall continue endlessly in the cycle of suffering and conflict. This is because we do not have a deep, internal understanding of the nature of karma. Those who do have this understanding never create negative actions with reckless abandon as we do. Whenever attachment or selfishness motivates our actions, even though we know full well that they are completely negative, we just go ahead and do them anyway.

I know Westerners quite well. They are intelligent, but their minds are split. On the one hand they desire to have perfect wisdom and to keep their karma straight. On the other they are impelled by the force of their bad habits, which prevents them from keeping their karma straight. This causes them much suffering. It even makes them cry! These people are very sensitive. When difficult circumstances arise, the negative energy overpowers the positive because they have never built up within themselves the force of good habits and because they lack deep, internal understanding of the nature of karma, or of cause and effect.

Some people might then say, "Oh, karma is experienced only by those who believe in it. Those who don't believe in karma don't experience its effects." Many Westerners have given me this argument. This is a completely wrong conception. The law of karma applies whether you believe in it or not. If you act in a certain way, you are sure to experience the appropriate result, just as surely as taking poison will make you sick—even though you might think that it is medicine that you are swallowing. Once you've created the karma to experience a certain result, that's where you're headed.

Cows, pigs, and scorpions have no idea of what is and what is not karma—no beliefs one way or the other—but they still have to live out their karma. Their every action is motivated by either greed, ignorance, or hatred, and each definitely brings its own result. Therefore, you must never think that karmic actions and reactions are only a Buddhist thing, a lama thing. Karma is a scientific law governing all physical and non-physical phenomena in the universe. It is extremely important for you to understand this.

When I teach about karma, I don't usually give technical explanations such as those found in Tibetan texts. I simply tell students to look at the way their minds are working at that very moment. They can easily see how up-and-down their minds really are, especially during a meditation course. Once they are aware of this problem, it is easy for them to understand how it has come from their previous experiences, and that karma is exactly that. It becomes clear to them without my having to use any new, technical terminology. Simply put, the uncontrolled body, speech, and mind are manifestations of karma.

Thus, we are all under the control of the true law of karma, whether we believe in it or not. Don't think that followers of Christianity, Judaism, and Islam are beyond the reach of karma and do not need to take care of it. It's not true. For example, Jews and Arabs have built up karma with each other, and now there are all sorts of problems in the Middle East. Butchers do not believe that their killing animals will have any negative repercussions, but whether they believe it or not, their giving such suffering to other beings will definitely come back upon them.

For instance, when you first come to Kathmandu you enjoy yourself and make yourself very comfortable. Then when you come up to Kopan Monastery, you feel agitated. You think it's very dirty and that there are no proper toilets.[3] Your agitation is the result of your previous attachment to comfort. That, too, is karma. If you weren't attached to your earlier experiences of comfort, you wouldn't care so much about your surroundings. Thus, you can get a clear understanding of karmic action and reaction simply by analyzing your everyday experiences.

I think this is a far better and more powerful way of developing mindfulness of your actions than by becoming obsessed, as so many Westerners are, with the cultivation of single-pointed concentration (*samadhi*) and insight meditation (*vipassana*). If that happens, you run the risk of thinking that sitting meditation is the only form of Dharma practice and that all other activities, such as eating, talking, and sleeping, are completely samsaric and negative. When you believe that these things are negative, they become negative.

What I'm saying is that there are many ways to meditate. Vipassana is not the only kind of meditation. Insight can be gained by meditating on any phenomenon in the universe. And you don't have to be sitting cross-legged to meditate: guarding your karma day in and day out is also meditation and can be a powerful way to develop insight. In this way your entire life can be used to bring you closer to the wisdom of egolessness.

When you understand the nature of karma, you are constantly aware of everything you do. Thus, wherever you go, you cannot escape from meditation. You know that if you do not maintain awareness of the actions of your body, speech, and mind, you will create one negativity after another and will have to experience the resultant suffering of confusion and dissatisfaction. This makes you conscious all the time: when dealing with others, eating in restaurants, shopping in a supermarket, or working at your job.

Usually our dualistic minds interpret the ordinary activities of daily life as being samsaric, dissatisfactory, suffering, and undesirable—impossible to use as objects for insight meditation. This is a gross misapprehension. Mahayana Buddhism teaches that if bodily sensations such as physical feelings can be used for the development of insight, so can any other form of sensory experience, such as the taste of food on the tongue.

Some people say that visualizations cannot be used for insight meditation because they are a mental projection, as if one's breath or feelings in the body were more real. Sensations and feelings are just as illusory as are visualizations of the Buddha. Bodily sensations are not permanent. They change from moment to moment because the relative mind is constantly changing. The feelings of the body and mind, especially those caused by the negative mind, are the projections of ignorance. Your dualistic mind automatically projects a dualistic view of whatever you experience.

Ordinary people who start to practice what they consider to be vipassana meditation believe that the world of bodily sensations is real. But no matter whether they use an internal or an external object of meditation, it still exists only in their imagination and in the view of their relative mind. Fundamentally, there is no difference between inner and outer phenomena: either both are true or both are hallucinations. Until you have realized non-duality, sunyata, whatever you experience, either physically or mentally, is an hallucinatory wrong view.

Actually, the taste of food on the tongue is also a bodily sensation. To think that it is not is a wrong conception. The Mahayana tradition contains meditation practices for every action. Tantric yoga teaches us that when we eat, we should first offer and bless the food. While eating, we should be relaxed and aware of whatever we are doing, constantly remembering the dependent nature of ourselves and the food, and not grasping at the sensory pleasure of eating, as we usually do. Any object can be used for the development of insight.

Mantra recitation can also be a great help in the practice of insight meditation. It makes the mind focus single-pointedly, thereby counteracting scattering and other distractions. However, the recitation does not have to be verbal. Mantra is a sound that has existed within your nervous system since before you were born, and is audible if you listen wisely. Mantra is not something that you receive, all of a sudden, from a lama. Without the natural vibration of sound within your nervous system, you would be deaf—each kind of energy has its own natural sound. This is not religious dogma, but something you can discover scientifically. You cannot abandon the natural sound of your nervous system. You might as well try to abandon your head!

However, it is the experience of countless lamas that the unstable, transitory objects of the five senses are more of a hindrance than a help in the development of single-pointed concentration. As long as you continue to perceive things with your relative mind and to grasp at objects of the five senses, you will not be able to realize single-pointed concentration. You will be neither a samadhi meditator nor a vipassana meditator. Check to see whether or not this is true.

Thus you can understand how ridiculous it is to think that sitting, trying to gain samadhi is the only way to practice Dharma, and that anything to do with living in the world is totally negative. You should constantly take care of every aspect of your life—waking, working, eating, sleeping—with understanding wisdom. Whether you are close to your guru, to the Sangha, to your parents, or all alone, you must take care of your karma as best you can. It is quite wrong to believe that you can outsmart karma by locking yourself in your room, thinking that when you are by yourself, you can do whatever you like. There is no escape! Whether you are with others or not, karmic reactions come automatically.

If we were to teach you that the only way to meditate was to sit and think of nothing, you would find no time to practice. Karma ensures that most Westerners have to spend their lives either working or doing other external activities. Since you couldn't find time to sit, you would think that your Dharma practice was history. But meditation is not blank-minded navel-gazing. When you have an understanding of the fundamentals of Dharma, you will see how much there is for you to do and how much you can grow. This gives you constant interest in maintaining your practice, and even though you cannot concentrate, you know that you can still practice Dharma. Wherever you go, whether you are with other practitioners or with worldly people, you know how to make your life one with Dharma. This ability comes from wisdom.

Without wisdom, how can you make the inescapable activities of eating, sleeping, and excreting one with Dharma? When you have wisdom, you don't always have to be around your guru to receive teachings. You can see the teachings in everything around you. You can learn from the movement of the planets, the weather, the growth and decay of plants, and all other phenomena. This is what happens when you have wisdom. In fact, your own wisdom understanding reality is your real guru. This is what Tibetan Buddhism teaches you.

Integrate your whole life with the experience of Dharma. That is the most powerful thing you can do. That is the way to reach enlightenment in one lifetime, because you do not waste a moment of your time. This is perfectly logical. If you believe the absolutely wrong conception that your one-hour daily meditation is the only chance you have to practice Dharma and that the other twenty-three hours of your day are completely dark, impure, and samsaric, you will definitely take three countless great eons to reach enlightenment! What your mind believes becomes reality for you, whether it is reality or not.

2

Taking Refuge

So far I have been talking about why we need purification and how it works. I have also emphasized that we have been unable to stop continuously creating negativities of body, speech, and mind because we have not yet understood the inner cause, the law of karma.

There is a big difference between a merely intellectual understanding of karma and one based on the living experience of how it works. Some students have word-perfect understanding of the teachings on karma and some superficial faith—"It must be true because my lama said so." But because they do not have any understanding of karma through experience, when their understanding is tested, they fail. They have no solution when serious problems arise. They are satisfied with being able to talk about karma, as if being able to tell their parents and friends all about it were enough, but they cannot *do* what they talk about because they haven't practiced.

Other students, however, are not satisfied with a merely intellectual understanding but prefer to understand through practice what they have been taught. They may not be able to give extensive discourses on karma, but because they are always mindful of their actions, they get a true taste of Dharma, an experience as real as the sweet taste of honey on your tongue. And when problems arise for such practitioners, they know how to apply the solutions. You must be clear about this. It is very dangerous to be content with just an intellectual understanding of Dharma and not to practice. That cannot help you.

Many Western and Eastern professors and scholars, who admit they don't practice, can speak at length on all aspects of Buddhist philosophy. Ask them a question and they can answer. But their explanations are like those of tourist guides—very superficial. When an experienced practitioner talks, his words have a blessed energy. He may be talking about the same thing that the scholars are, but the way he expresses himself touches your heart. The talk of those without experience is like the empty wind whistling about your ears.

If you understand cause and effect through your own experience, there is no way you can be careless in anything you do. Although those whose knowledge is merely intellectual can express their conceptual understanding of karma in perfect language and give lectures to huge gatherings of people, they do not really believe what they are talking about because they have not tasted the honey of what they know. They do not live by the ethics they discuss. Personally, I find this rather painful. When asked a practical question about how karma works, these scholars can answer only by quoting some book or text they have read. Since they have no experience, they cannot explain precisely how to observe karma, what to do in practice, and how observing karma leads your mind in a positive direction. Some practical questions go beyond the scholars' philosophical framework of karma, and so they can't relate to them. All they can say is, "You can't ask that question. Buddhism doesn't deal with that." That's not the way it is.

I am sure that most of you understand clearly how defiled actions of body, speech, and mind are cyclic in nature, bringing the results of suffering, confusion, and more defilement. In your minds there is no question about the truth of this. You can probably explain it much more clearly than I can. When you hear my broken English, you think to yourselves, "What kind of language is that! If only he'd let me talk, I could give a much better explanation." All this is true. But why can't you put a stop to your negative habits? Theoretical knowledge alone is not enough.

Many Buddhists with little learning have attained high spiritual realizations through acting seriously at a practical level. Many great scholars who can lecture at length have reached nowhere. Therefore, I advise you to be careful. When you talk about the teachings it is not what you say but how you have gained your knowledge that is important. Your speech must carry the blessed vibration of personal experience and convey that energy to your listeners.

In Tibet, when skillful, realized lamas gave teachings on the graduated path to enlightenment, often they would not emphasize philosophical doctrine but the practical aspects of the teaching; they would even make the students meditate while they taught. As a result, some students would receive realizations during the discourse. By the end of a twenty-day teaching, they would understand the entire path from beginning to end and, full of energy, would want to rush off from the monastery into mountain caves for long meditation retreats. On the other hand, scholars could teach you the same subject for twenty years without touching your heart.

I have also seen Westerners so energized by the lam-rim teachings that they too have wanted to rush off into the mountains. However, continuous practice over many years is a much more powerful way of purifying negative actions and much better for you than impulsive, emotional bursts of meditation in solitary retreat.

Thus, when you take refuge and generate bodhicitta, there should be no gap between them and your own mind. If refuge and bodhicitta are not one with your mind, they cannot purify the negativities we discussed before. When you take refuge, your mind should be one with refuge; when you generate bodhicitta, your mind should become bodhicitta. It should not be that you are sitting down *here* on your cushion, dualistically doing something out *there* in front of you. Your mind should become the Dharma that you practice. It is difficult but possible, and it is essential if your practice is to benefit your mind.

Because Westerners not only listen but act, many students at our Kopan courses on the graduated path to enlightenment have had strong positive experiences. These students were sincere and sensitive and communicated well with Lama Zopa and myself; their minds were influenced by what they heard. If in a teaching situation the teacher is just like a radio and the audience like the walls of a room, how can there be any benefit? Furthermore, the natural skepticism of Westerners that does not allow them to accept what they hear until they understand it makes them exceptionally well qualified to listen to Mahayana teachings. I like it when they say, "You said so-and-so. I don't accept that." For example, we feel that those who have guru devotion based on emotional faith instead of understanding wisdom are not properly qualified to take teachings.

TAKING REFUGE AND GENERATING BODHICITTA

Forever, I take refuge in Buddha, Dharma, and Sangha, and in the Sangha of the three vehicles, the dakas and dakinis of secret mantra yoga, the heroes and heroines, the gods and goddesses, the bodhisattvas and, in particular, my guru.

"Vehicle" is the way we translate the Sanskrit word *yana.* Its connotation is that certain actions will definitely elevate your consciousness to a higher level. For example, if you cultivate bodhicitta and practice the six transcendental perfections, you will definitely achieve enlightenment. The Great Vehicle, the Mahayana, carries you from the beginning, bodhicitta, through the six transcendental perfections and the ten bodhisattva levels to the goal, enlightenment. If you begin perfectly and act correctly, your vehicle will definitely carry you to your desired destination. Yana also has the connotation of "path": the right path will lead you to the right place. If, out of ignorance, you follow the wrong path, you will get lost.

The three Buddhist vehicles are the two Hinayana vehicles and the one Mahayana, and we take refuge in the Sangha of all three. Even though we are following the Mahayana and, in particular, its profoundest aspect of tantric yoga, we should not be arrogant, thinking: "I'm a Mahayanist; I don't need to take refuge in the Hinayana Sangha." Although the Hinayana arhats do have some attachment to their own liberation, they have transcended their egos with full realization of sunyata and can guide us from samsara. Therefore, without discrimination, we take refuge in all Sangha.

Hinayana and Mahayana were not invented by Tibetan lamas. These two Buddhist schools were founded by the Buddha himself and were thus in existence long before the teachings arrived in Tibet. Some people think that the Buddha taught only in Pali and that sutras recorded in other languages are false. Others believe the same of Sanskrit. All such ideas are wrong. When the Dharma spread to other countries, realized practitioners, while retaining the essence of the teachings, adapted them to the minds of the people of their own country for the purposes of clear communication. After all, there are great differences between Tibetans from the snowy mountains and Indians from the hot plains, so you would expect some changes in the mode of expression of the Dharma when it went to one place from the other.

Once, a king who was a disciple of the Buddha had a dream in which eighteen people were fighting over a roll of cloth, each trying to get it for himself. Finally, each person finished up with a complete roll. The king went to the Buddha and asked him what it meant. He told the king that the roll of cloth symbolized his teaching and that the dream meant that after the Buddha's death, eighteen schools, each with its own, slightly different interpretation of his philosophy, would develop. Each person's receiving a complete roll meant that each of these schools would contain the correct, complete path to liberation. Thus, the establishment of the eighteen Hinayana schools was prophesied by the Buddha.

The Theravadin school is one of the eighteen. Some followers of the Hinayana feel insulted when they are called "Hinayanists" and insist on being called "Theravadins" (which doesn't make much sense, because as only one of the schools, Theravada does not contain the entire Hinayana philosophy, and thus, the two terms are not equivalent). And then again, there are others whose egos swell with pride when they think of themselves as "Mahayanists." Such dualistic reactions arise from ignorance and are entirely contrary to the inner peace of Dharma wisdom.

The main difference between Hinayanists and Mahayanists lies in their state of mind. The principal concern of a follower of the Hinayana is his own liberation; that of a follower of the Mahayana is the enlightenment of all sentient beings. Some may feel that wearers of yellow robes are Hinayanists and wearers of red, Mahayanists, but such superficial categorizations are usually wrong. Those who live by the great enthusiastic determination to lead all sentient beings to supreme enlightenment by themselves alone, giving not a thought to their own liberation, are Mahayanists, no matter what they wear. If those robed in red, overwhelmed by insight into the suffering and confusion of their own samsaric existence, are motivated solely by the wish to liberate themselves, giving no thought to the problems of others in samsara, they are Hinayanists.

We take refuge in the Mahayana as well as the Hinayana Sangha: dakas, dakinis, heroes, heroines, gods, goddesses, and bodhisattvas—all those who have realizations of the completion stage of highest yoga tantra. Some of these have a peaceful aspect; others appear wrathful.

Bodhisattvas do manifest wrathfully; you should not think that they always have to look peaceful. Even on the first of the ten bodhisattva levels, which is called the "Joyous One," they can manifest simultaneously in one hundred different bodies. With these they can take teachings directly from the *sambhogakaya* aspects of one hundred different buddhas or transform into one hundred different manifestations for the benefit of sentient beings. As bodhisattvas progress, their abilities increase tenfold with each level; what they can do is beyond our comprehension. Thus, bodhisattvas manifest in the aspect of peaceful and wrathful dakas, dakinis, and so forth, and we take refuge in them.

Actually, bodhisattvas can manifest as Easterners or Westerners, as dark- or light-skinned people, as Christians, Muslims, or Jews—in any aspect whatsoever. These days, many so-called religious people are narrow-minded. They would not go for spiritual guidance to a teacher whose race, gender, skin color, or nationality was different. When they align themselves with a particular guru, they become partial, believing that all other gurus and their followers are evil. I call this "guruism." That's wrong; it's taking refuge in a dualistic way. That is not the Buddhist way of taking refuge.

Of course, some so-called gurus claim that they are the best and only guru in the world, and their disciples naturally believe this. In this way, instead of becoming a vehicle for liberation, the religion they teach suffocates their followers, who become narrower and narrower, and end up as fanatics. It would be better to be non-religious than to finish up like this. At least non-religious people don't have such extreme views; for them, simply being human is enough.

We take refuge in the buddhas and bodhisattvas of the ten directions, in whoever has the realization of sunyata, no matter what their color, nationality, or creed. Remember, a first-level bodhisattva can be an African man or woman, a Saudi Arabian camel driver, perhaps even a terrorist, taking such a role to serve others better.

Finally—but, as it says in the prayer, in particular—we take refuge in our guru, especially our root guru, who has shown us the blissful path to the everlasting realization of enlightenment. Remember always that your guru is completely one with Heruka Vajrasattva. *Lob-pön* means the one who shows us the true path and guides us along it, straightening the actions of our body, speech, and mind and leading us away from blind, ignorant actions. He can lead us to enlightenment in one lifetime, or even in three years. Recalling our guru's inconceivable kindness, we take refuge in him forever.

The visualization we use when taking refuge is as follows. Your father is to your right, your mother, to your left. Your worst enemy, the sentient being who agitates you the most, is in front of you. Your dearest friend, the person to whom you are most attached, is placed behind you. All other sentient beings surround you on all sides.

This visualization is a good example of Mahayana psychology. If we were asked where we would like to put our best friend, we would normally say, "Oh, here! In front of me!" Similarly, we would prefer to put our enemy behind us, out of sight. Instead, when we take refuge we put our enemy right in front. Look at him or her; examine his or her life sincerely. Think of the problems that your own uncontrolled mind causes, and realize that your enemy is in exactly the same predicament. Analyze the way you feel toward this person.

"I think he is the worst person on earth, but his problems are the same as mine. Why should I feel angry whenever I see his face? The main thing wrong with him is his ego-grasping ignorance. If I'm going to be angry with anything, that's what I should be angry with. But his ignorant mind is invisible to my sense perceptions, so why do I react to his physical appearance? His body is merely the agent of his negative mind. His negative mind is the actual source of everything I don't like about him. May he realize this, purify his ignorance completely, and receive perfect realizations."

Thus, you should generate great compassion for your enemy and, with that, take refuge. This is the best way of taking refuge.

The practice of taking refuge in this way is itself a solution to your problems of ignorance, attachment, and hatred. Otherwise, you run the risk of being too worried about your own problems, and your taking refuge becomes simply a new way of augmenting your self-attachment and concern for your own realizations. You will say that you are practicing Dharma, but the Dharma that you practice will be nothing but another means of increasing your attachment. Because of your attitude, Dharma wisdom will become just one more material possession instead of the solution to your problems. Then, if someone says, "Your Dharma is *kaka*," your ego will explode in rage.

Wisdom is wisdom. Why should it bother you if some ignoramus tells you it is excrement or calls your lama a demon? You cannot make things into excrement and demons simply by calling them that! Therefore, be careful. If you get upset when someone criticizes your Dharma practice, it means that you have made Dharma wisdom into something material. This applies not only to Buddhism but to all other religions as well. If the followers of any religion are angered by someone's telling them that their religion is no good and they want to burn their critics at the stake, then their conceptions are completely wrong. Check now how you would react to such abuse—once you're angry, it's too late to check.

Visualizing all mother sentient beings around you while taking refuge is a very powerful means of overcoming excessive concern for your own problems. Many of us are too obsessed with our own problems. We cannot forget them and never think of what others are experiencing. When we finally realize that others have exactly the same troubles that we do, we start to feel, "I'm not the worst person in the world after all; nor am I alone in my suffering. There are many just like me. I should have exactly the same sort of compassion for them as I do for myself."

How do the Buddha, the Dharma, and the three vehicles' Sangha save us from the confusion of samsara? It depends on our mental attitude. We have to understand the nature of our samsaric existence and the great power and ability those holy beings have to guide us out of it. "I am truly helpless. Although I am intelligent enough to make my life comfortable and even enjoyable, I do not have the knowledge or wisdom to overcome the gravitational pull of my attachment to sense pleasures that binds me to samsara. There is no way I can free myself from this. But those holy beings can really guide me. They have the method, the solution, the light of wisdom to dispel my ignorance, the key to open my mind so that knowledge-wisdom can grow. I am so tired of always being uncontrolled, of endlessly going on and on. The buddhas show the perfect way from darkness into light. The Sangha guides me and all others from our confusion. And Dharma wisdom is the actual guide, the true path and the true cessation of suffering."

There are many levels of meaning in the word *Dharma*, as I am sure you have learned from your sutra studies. When you take refuge in Dharma, your actual object of refuge is the wisdom that fully understands absolute nature and is completely one with sunyata, totally free from dualistic view. We always talk about Dharma, but what is Dharma? Dharma is wisdom—Dharma wisdom. However, it takes a long time and the accumulation of many realizations to attain the ultimate wisdom. We have to work at this. To run properly, an automobile depends upon many parts, none of which is the complete automobile itself. Similarly, perfect wisdom is composed of many different sorts of knowledge, each of which is an integral part of the path of wisdom.

Thus, you can understand that there is a difference between the

Dharma refuge we are talking about here—perfect wisdom, which fully understands absolute nature, sunyata—and the usual Dharma we discuss—the wisdom solution to mental problems. That perfect wisdom is the ultimate object of refuge. Many of my students complain that they have been waiting in vain for me to teach sunyata. But you see—here I have been teaching it all along. It is just that I did not call it sunyata: "Come here; I'll show you sunyata! Tomorrow you'll reach enlightenment!" I have been camouflaging it in simpler terms.

The buddhas show you the Dharma and how it works within you to bring the true cessation of suffering. Through putting it into practice you become a buddha. The Sangha help you to create the right conditions for practice and make sure that you purify your negativities and gain true cessation. As I said before, bodhisattvas manifest in numberless ways for the sole purpose of helping us in our practice. When they show a wrathful aspect, we should not get upset and think that they no longer love us. Instead we should think, "This bodhisattva is showing me how awful I look when I'm angry. If he hadn't done that, I would never have known. I should be grateful for his kindness." Whenever anybody is angry with us, we should think that he or she is a manifestation of a bodhisattva teaching us not to be angry. Similarly, whenever anybody around us is very peaceful, we should think with joy that this person too is a bodhisattva, showing us that others get much pleasure when we behave well.

You must have noticed that the moment you see certain people you feel happy, but with others you immediately feel uncomfortable. This is karma at work. Within you there is some energy that causes this to happen; there is almost nothing you can do about it. Handsome men and beautiful women are spontaneously treated well wherever they go; ugly ones are treated badly. This is their karma: even though they don't want it, it is very difficult to change. What kind of scientific explanation are Westerners going to offer for this common phenomenon? Karma makes your life difficult; karma makes it easy.

However, this is not to say that karma is permanent or fixed. Karma is a changeable phenomenon. All the same, until the energy of a certain karma is expended, one has to tolerate one's situation.

Take, for example, Gomchen, the monastery dog. We all love him; Lord Buddha loves him; Jesus loves him, too. Despite all this, no one can communicate with him in order to show him the absolute nature, sunyata.

Until his body changes into a more suitable one it will be impossible to have this sort of contact with him. That is his karma. All samsaric sentient beings have to accept what they are going through until the power of the karmic energy behind that experience has run out. Everything in your life depends upon this kind of energy. When the causal energy of a particular action is exhausted, it can no longer bring an effect. Examine your life; in this way you can understand karma. Each sentient being lives according to his or her own way of thinking, level of conscious energy, attitude, and environment. That is karma. I am using the word *karma* a lot here. I hope you understand what I mean.

In conclusion, then, all buddhas show you the true path and true cessation, the Dharma that liberates you from samsara. And they try to make you realize that what really guides you is your acting correctly, in accordance with the path. This means that you, not the buddhas, are ultimately responsible for your own liberation. You have to understand this clearly.

The Sangha of the three vehicles, including protectors such as Mahakala and Kalarupa, are your friends; they help you whenever they can. Thus, you should know what Sangha really means. Most people think that Sangha refers to those who have taken robes, but there's no text that says that only those in robes are Sangha. However, we *can* say that those who have dedicated their lives to Dharma by taking ordination are *relative* Sangha. The ultimate Sangha are those who have the perfect realization of absolute nature, sunyata, in their minds; irrespective of the clothes they wear, the color of their skin, or anything else, they are the real Sangha, your best friends.

You often feel lonely, but you never should. Your true, everlasting Sangha friends are always with you: the dakas and dakinis, the peaceful and wrathful bodhisattvas, and the other Sangha of the three vehicles. They can guide you from worldly agitation and confusion. When you realize this you will never miss friends or feel alone. Meditate; go within: that's where your real friends are.

VISUALIZING THE OBJECT OF REFUGE

The way we take refuge in the Heruka Vajrasattva practice is different from the way we do it according to the teachings on the graduated path to enlightenment, where the principal refuge object is Shakyamuni

Buddha. Here the Buddha refuge object can be either Heruka or Vajradhara, whichever is easier for you to visualize.

Visualize a standing blue Heruka, embracing his consort, red Vajra Varahi. Around them are many dakas and dakinis, the sixty-two deities of the Heruka mandala, and countless buddhas, bodhisattvas, and arhats, who have attained the realization of everlasting peace.

If you prefer to visualize Vajradhara, he is seated in the full lotus position embracing his consort, Vajradhatu Ishvari (Tib. Ying-chug-ma). Again, he is blue and she is red, and they are surrounded by the same manifestations of divine wisdom as before, except for the sixty-two deities of the Heruka mandala. However, whether you visualize Heruka or Vajradhara, remember that it is actually your guru appearing in that aspect; that the deity you visualize as the principal object of refuge is completely one with your guru. Thus Heruka (or Vajradhara) is Buddha; the dakas, dakinis, and other Sangha of the three vehicles are Sangha; and their wisdom is Dharma.

One benefit of visualizing Heruka in the standing position is that it blesses your nervous system and activates the kundalini energy within it. This helps your practice of maha-anuttara yoga tantra.

Visualizations are not objects of the eye consciousness; you cannot see them by staring in front of you. Heruka's divine body is a manifestation of his divine transcendental wisdom, which transforms into that divine form and appears instantaneously in the space in front of you. Since this visualization is a transformation of and one with the blissful omniscient mind, it is in the nature of consciousness. We cannot perceive divine transcendental wisdom through the eye or our other physical senses. Thus, in order to communicate with us, the energy of the ultimate wisdom manifests in this profound, clean-clear divine form, which is in the nature of light. Also, it does not appear gradually but with the suddenness of a movie instantly projected onto the screen, or a person suddenly appearing in a doorway. Through visualizations such as this we can easily communicate with the *dharmakaya.*

After you have taken refuge, the Buddhas and the Sangha of the three vehicles—the dakas and dakinis, peaceful and wrathful bodhisattvas, protectors such as Mahakala and Kalarupa, and so forth—melt into light and dissolve into the principal deity, Heruka. Vajra Varahi also becomes light and absorbs into Heruka. Finally, Heruka himself melts into light that dissolves into his heart. This ball of light comes to the crown of your head and descends through your central channel, passing through your throat chakra to melt into your heart chakra. You become absolutely one with this light, which is in essence Heruka and your guru. Remain concentrated on that for as long as you can, without allowing dualistic thoughts of *this* and *that* to disturb you.

With practice, you might be able to remain in this single-pointed concentration on non-dual oneness for half an hour. When wrong conceptions begin to arise, leave this meditation and generate bodhicitta:

I must become Heruka in order to lead all sentient beings to the sublime state of Heruka-hood.

THE THREE WAYS OF TAKING REFUGE

There are three ways of taking refuge: outer, inner, and secret. Most people think that the sutra, or *Paramitayana,* way of taking refuge is the only one. This is what we call outer refuge and is the method usually explained when teachings on refuge are given. In outer refuge, the Buddha in whom we take refuge is somebody other than ourselves: a person who has attained buddhahood, an enlightened being such as Shakyamuni Buddha. The Dharma refuge in this system is the teaching given by that enlightened being. The outer Sangha comprises the ordained or realized followers of the Dharma teachings, as I explained before. Understanding that the already-existent Buddha, Dharma, and Sangha have the power to guide us, and fearing the sufferings of samsara, we take refuge in them.

The other two ways of taking refuge are methods of tantric yoga. Inner refuge is taking refuge in the buddha you yourself will become. The wisdom of that, your own future buddha, is the inner Dharma refuge object. When you have attained that state, you yourself become Sangha: that is the inner Sangha refuge object. At that stage, you not only become Sangha, you attain unity with all Three Jewels of refuge and no longer have to take refuge in something separate from yourself.

When you take inner refuge, your mind becomes transcendental omniscient wisdom; this transforms into the divine aspect of Heruka (or Vajradhara), along with the dakas and dakinis, the peaceful and wrathful bodhisattvas, and so forth, and you take refuge in that. To do this you need to have at least a deep intellectual understanding of the false conceptions and projections of your ego so that you can somehow purify these at the moment of taking refuge. You can see that this is quite difficult.

Secret refuge is the third way of taking refuge. This way of taking refuge is the most difficult of all. You have to recognize that your nervous system is pervaded by blissful daka-dakini energy instead of the usual ridiculous energy of gravitational attachment to sense pleasures, and you take refuge in that. Here you are utilizing your nervous system's energy resources to generate simultaneously born great bliss, which you unify with the wisdom of non-duality, taking it as the blissful path to liberation. This experience is really what liberates you from dissatisfaction and dualistic concepts. Most people are not aware of the blissful energy that lies within themselves. But when they create the right situation through practices such as this yoga method or *tum-mo* meditation, for example, they can experience an explosion of blissful energy that they would never have thought possible.[4] I also heard recently that some people experienced incredible blissful energy within their nervous systems while doing the fasting retreat with my *chu-len* pills.[5]

These three ways of taking refuge are entirely non-contradictory and have been taught so that practitioners can choose the method that best suits their level of mental development. Outer refuge is for the least developed, secret refuge for the fortunate, highly intelligent few.

If you understand the true meaning of taking refuge, you will know what a positive effect it has on your mind and experience its great benefits. You will really enjoy taking refuge, and every time you do, the pure energy of your innermost heart will grow. If you do not know how to take refuge properly, whatever meditation you do will be like snow on the road, which looks very impressive as it falls, but quickly disappears. Like that, your meditation will have no lasting effect. With a deep understanding of taking refuge, you will begin to taste the honey of Lord Buddha's wisdom.

3

Inner Refuge and Meditation on Emptiness

Understanding Sunyata

Why is the practice of inner refuge emphasized by tantric yoga so difficult? Because it is mainly done by the mind. To begin with, refuge has to be taken from the heart. It is not something superficial where you just repeat a few words while your mind remains unmoved. Some people take refuge as a social custom. They chant "Namo gurubhya, namo buddhaya, namo dharmaya, namo sanghaya" with no understanding of the practice or the meaning of the words and no change in their minds. Others chant the refuge formula "Namo gurubhya..." just because they are with other people who are reciting it. That is not taking refuge—it has no more to do with the path to liberation than eating breakfast every morning or going to church on Sundays out of ingrained habit or social obligation.

As I mentioned above, when we take inner refuge, our mind should become the wisdom of the greatest transcendental bliss and transform into the divine aspect of Heruka. Then we take refuge. Do not look outside for the object of refuge! I know you will think it should be somewhere out in front of you. That is your dualistic way of thinking: "*I* am taking *refuge*." *You* are sitting down *here*, doing *something* out *there*. Your dualistic mind immediately discriminates between subject and object. As soon as you think you are doing something you automatically think of external activities. This happens because you have so many dualistic imprints on your mind.

So, when taking inner refuge, your mind itself becomes the greatest blissful transcendental wisdom. While you generate great faith in and devotion to that wisdom, it simultaneously transforms and appears to you as Heruka. Feeling completely one with Heruka, you take refuge. This psychological method is extremely beneficial. It may be hard to understand, but you should try.

To be able to understand this way of taking refuge we have to understand sunyata. If we do not, the transformation of our minds into the greatest, everlasting, blissful transcendental wisdom becomes just a dry intellectual concept instead of a powerful inner experience. If we have a proper understanding of the absolute nature—if our minds have been touched by the experience of sunyata—it is relatively easy for our minds to become the greatest transcendental wisdom, to transform into Heruka, and for us to feel oneness with this. In this way our minds mix with the transcendental blissful energy of Heruka instead of the usual hatred, desire, and attachment.

If your mind is truly mixed with the great transcendental blissful energy of divine wisdom, you do not need to say the words of the refuge prayer, "Namo gurubhya...." Words are not refuge. All the same, weak people do need words as a way of communicating; words have some meaning for them. But if you have the realization of the constant, blissful feeling of oneness, you do not have to take refuge with your mouth. Wherever you go, whatever you do, you are taking refuge all the time; because of your constant faith, your very being is in the nature of refuge. You know that the everlasting, blissful transcendental wisdom is most profound, most pure. Whenever you eat, whenever you drink, your mind is one with the blissful energy of Heruka, so you are always taking refuge. Taking refuge does not mean sitting cross-legged in meditation. Thus you make constant progress on the path no matter what you are doing, and in that way, can quickly reach enlightenment.

The realization of sunyata has the quality of everlasting joy. Samsaric pleasures, on the other hand, are transitory and painful: here one minute, gone the next. Because they suddenly disappear, they cause us pain. If we weren't attached to samsaric pleasures, we wouldn't be hurt when they disappeared.

If we do not have a perfect understanding of sunyata through realization, we should at least have a clear conceptual knowledge of it, in order to overcome the wrong conception of the way we exist, which is deeply imprinted upon our consciousness. The ordinary, relative idea we have of ourselves is very physical. I think, "I am Thubten Yeshe," and in my mind there is this extremely thick image of a head, arms, legs, and grasping sense organs. As long as you see yourself like this you cannot mix your consciousness with the everlasting, blissful transcendental wisdom. An understanding of sunyata automatically causes this ordinary, relative image to disappear.

If you have sharp intelligence it is not so difficult to understand sunyata. You do not have to learn tremendously complex philosophies or study volumes of texts under many lamas. Of course, you *can* learn from teachers and books, but if you are skillful, you can learn through a very simple method: do not believe what your senses tell you. It is not necessary to search far and wide for what stops you from seeing sunyata. Simply realize that the way you perceive the sense world every day of your life is completely wrong, that it is the misconceived projection of your ego. The moment you realize this, your deluded view will disappear. One reason that the yoga method is so powerful is that it allows you to see very quickly how your ego's projections are wrong and to cut through them completely.

We often feel insecure. On the way to meet someone we think, "Maybe she won't like me," "Maybe he won't like me," "I wish I were better looking," "Maybe she won't like the way I speak," and things like that. All such insecure thoughts derive from wrong conceptions and misinterpretations. As soon we realize that everything has been painted by our ignorant mind, that our illusory views, thoughts, and feelings are not even relatively true, let alone absolutely, we shall stop feeling insecure. Even if others abuse us, call us thieves and the like, we'll have control and won't suffer. Such are the practical benefits of this kind of understanding.

We live in the sense world believing that the misconceptions and projections of our ignorant mind are true. We think that seeing is believing: "I saw that; it must be true." Some people believe passionately that their philosophy is the ideal one for their society. Communist or capitalist, both are wrong; both are hallucinations! If we go on like this, we shall never discover sunyata; it will always be somewhere else. When we realize that our view of the world is a hallucination, that our view of reality is obscured by the heavy blanket of delusion, the wrong view disappears, and we are left with its opposite, the right view of sunyata. The moment we extinguish the dualistic mind, we experience sunyata.

Thus, you can study sunyata every day, because every day your five senses' gravitational attachment to the sense world has you believing that whatever you perceive really exists as it appears. If you continuously investigate your perceptions and beliefs, there is no time that you are not studying sunyata. Sometimes books and philosophies can be more of a hindrance than a help in your understanding of sunyata, because if you do not know how to integrate words with experience, they can cause conflict in your mind. If you *do* know how to do this, then even one word can become a great teaching for you.

Those who think that understanding sunyata necessitates studying vast numbers of scriptures and committing to memory thousands of words of text are liable to get discouraged. They feel that trying to understand sunyata in their lifetime is a hopeless task. But you can easily understand sunyata by realizing that your ignorant mind's view of any object is completely illusory, not even relatively existent, even though for countless lives your ego-grasping and self-attachment have made you believe "this is really this" and "that is really that," and caused you great suffering. As long as your mind is ignorant, you will perceive any object dualistically. Any object perceived in that way is actually non-existent.

However, you cannot say that nothing exists: "My nose, my tongue, my mouth—nothing of me exists." How can you say that there is no light, no table? This form of intellectual negation is completely wrong. Better, investigate whether or not *your view* of a table really exists. You will find that it definitely does not. Investigate your views of anything—you will find that none of them exist as they appear. You always say things like, "Nepal is like this," "America is like that," "Europe is like this." You are talking nonsense. The Nepal, America, and Europe you are talking about do not exist. You think, "Oh, this meditation course is too heavy," or "This retreat is such suffering." You are living in a dream world of dream projections. Your dreaming mind is making you suffer.

All the same, this does not mean that you can deny the existence of the sense world. That is totally illogical. You should not concern yourself with whether Nepal exists or not; your business is to discover whether your mind's interpretation of Nepal exists or not. The problem is that your wrong conceptions build up a view of Nepal that has nothing whatsoever to do with the true nature of Nepal, even relatively, and you cling to it. My ignorant mind builds up its view, "Thubten Yeshe is like this, like this, like this"—which has nothing whatsoever to do with my true nature—and I cling with attachment to this unreal, self-pitying projection. Sentient beings have developed attachment over countless lives because they believe that without something to cling to they are lost. When sentient beings *believe* they are lost, they really get lost. For example, during the death process they panic in terror because they feel they are losing everything.

To realize the right view, sunyata, first you have to search for and discover it within your own mind. If you start by searching for ultimate nature in external phenomena, such as trees, tables, and other persons, you will never find it. In the experience of the great Indian pandits and Tibetan lamas, sunyata can never be found like that.

Samsaric beings are by nature very outward looking. We always think that we can understand reality by looking at what other people are doing. We try to assess our own progress by checking out our neighbors. What do they possess? How did they get it? This approach itself makes it impossible to find reality. If this is your attitude, you'll never find sunyata, even if you study it your whole life.

To discover our inner nature, to have the inner realization of sunyata, we must begin by searching for the absolute nature of our own minds. When we have discovered reality within, it will be much easier to discover the reality of external phenomena. The principal means of realizing sunyata is not through intellectual exercises, such as studying the words of other teachers or engaging in logical debate. Through such methods alone we cannot discover sunyata. We also have to investigate our own minds to identify our wrong concepts and views and practice methods of purification.

Why have we not yet discovered the ultimate nature, sunyata, that lies within our minds, even though we may have studied it for years? Because the vibration of mental defilements and impurities prevents us from doing so. Therefore, to allow sunyata wisdom to grow within us, it is very important that while we study the teachings on sunyata and investigate our minds, we cleanse these hindering negativities through purifying methods, such as prostrations and the Vajrasattva yoga method. In other words, to make progress in understanding sunyata in order to fully realize it, we must do two things: develop our intellectual understanding of sunyata and purify our mental hindrances, including the wrong concepts and views we have discovered through analyzing our minds. The power of this combined approach will make it much easier for us to realize sunyata.

Once, the great Tibetan teacher Lama Tsong Khapa was studying and analyzing sunyata according to the teachings of the Madhyamaka school, when Manjushri appeared to him and said, "At this point, nobody on earth can teach you sunyata." So Lama Tsong Khapa went to an isolated place, made powerful purification, and meditated, and in that way finally received direct, non-conceptual knowledge of sunyata according to the view of Nagarjuna's Middle Way philosophy. Thus the yoga method of Heruka Vajrasattva is not solely for purifying negativities but is also a method for making possible the quick discovery of the ultimate nature, sunyata, within our minds through its powerful destruction of wrong conceptions.

This long discussion on sunyata has come about from the explanation of inner refuge. To take inner refuge properly, we must understand sunyata and purify the wrong view of ourselves projected by our ego. The moment we start to think, "I am so-and-so, born there, brought up like this...," problems begin. Our ego's projections are a natural source of problems. For example, when someone is born into a Jewish family, he identifies with the Jewish race, and thousands of years of historical problems come to him. As long as there's ego, there will automatically be problems.

The marvelous quality of Lord Buddha's psychology is that it can eradicate all problems and their cause completely and forever. In this it is the exact opposite of Western psychology, which merely alleviates symptoms; as the root of problems is left intact, the removal of one set of symptoms simply results in the growth of another. We should understand and appreciate the psychological mechanism by which Lord Buddha's yoga method works in the treatment of human problems.

When you actualize the evolutionary yoga method and generate yourself in the divine form of the deity, you should understand that it works through the power of your wisdom of sunyata. It is absolutely nothing like your becoming, for example, a candle. The two things are completely different. You must be really clear about this; it is very dangerous if you are not. I think Western understanding of this process has a long way to go. You must understand the difference.

When you understand sunyata, you have the power to bring your mind into oneness with the blissful transcendental wisdom that is totally beyond projections of ego. That wisdom transforms into the deity. You can see what a vast difference there is between your becoming Heruka

Vajrasattva and your becoming a candle! If you do not have a deep understanding of how the evolutionary yoga method works, then when somebody disputes your practice—"What's the difference between becoming Heruka Vajrasattva and becoming a candle? You'd be better off becoming a rose. At least you'd smell good!"—you have no answer. You start to doubt what you are doing: "That's a powerful argument. I have no answer. Perhaps my whole practice has no greater benefit than trying to become a candle." If this is the level of your understanding of the practice, it is less than nothing. You must know the difference.

Most of you practice meditations where you have to visualize Shakyamuni Buddha or a deity such as Avalokiteshvara. If you have at least an intellectual understanding of sunyata, you find visualization easy. If you do not, your wrong conceptions project in such a physical way that it is very difficult for you to visualize the divine wisdom transforming from sunyata into the divine form of the deity. On the other hand, if you are aware that the all-embracing divine wisdom of the buddhas is everywhere, your understanding faith makes it easy for you to visualize the divine form of the Buddha suddenly appearing in the space in front of you. As I explained before, the full visualization appears at once: you do not have to start with a baby Buddha that gradually grows to completion.

Thus, the way of taking refuge in the practice of tantric yoga is not easy. It is much more difficult than taking outer refuge as explained in the sutra teachings on the graduated path to enlightenment. However, once your mind has reached a certain stage of development, you can definitely practice inner refuge. Also, you should understand that these different ways of taking refuge are not contradictory. The tantric yoga method is not implying that the sutra method is no good, or wrong. These different methods have been taught because people's minds are at different stages of development. At this time I do not think it is necessary to give any further explanation of secret refuge.

GENERATING BODHICITTA

After meditating on refuge, we generate bodhicitta according to the methods of tantric yoga. This means feeling the greatest enthusiasm for reaching Heruka-hood quickly—as quickly as possible—so that we can lead all mother sentient beings to Heruka-hood in the shortest possible time. If we feel like this we can never be lazy.

For example, what if your dear mother were caught in a blazing fire. You would not relax and say, "Let her burn. I don't have time to get her out right now. I'll do it later." Of course you would stop whatever you were doing at the time, no matter how important, and immediately rush to rescue her without wasting a moment. Similarly, when you realize that mother sentient beings are trapped and burning in the fire of wrong conceptions and negativities, there is no way to be lazy. You have to transform every action of your life—eating, sleeping, working—into Dharma wisdom. You cannot allow yourself to lapse into samsaric behavior for even a moment.

But we *are* lazy. Our impure mind lets us live life as if it were a tea party: "Let my mother burn—I'll pull her out of the fire when I've finished enjoying myself." Of course, we do not say these words, but our inner feeling, beyond words, reflects this attitude. Be careful; we often behave like this. Imagine: I'm at a first-class restaurant having a good time, when all of a sudden one of my students comes rushing in to tell me that my mother is in flames. I just sit there and reply, "Later; I have a dessert to finish!" I mean, you'd want to beat me for my selfishness, wouldn't you? Of course, this is a bit of an exaggeration, but it shows the sort of attitude we have.

All the same, we should not get emotional about all this. If I pump you up too much, you'll get over-excited and not want to do anything but run off to the mountains to meditate. That becomes another problem. I am not trying to excite you; it is much better to have calm, understanding wisdom. As I mentioned before, often in Tibet, after lam-rim teachings, the students would be so full of energy that all they wanted to do was leave their studies at the monastery and rush off into the mountains, to live and meditate like Milarepa. Actually, many of them did go, but of course, most of them came back a few days later.

Nevertheless, this shows how powerful the Dharma can be. Sometimes people feel that the lamas are powerful, they change your life. But it is Dharma wisdom that changes the human mind. Dharma wisdom comes into your consciousness, and your mental attitudes change. That is the power of the Dharma, not the magic of the lamas. We don't even know any magic!

When you practice the sadhana of Heruka Vajrasattva, the refuge and bodhicitta prayers are recited three times. Why these repetitions? To ensure that you have time to meditate and imbue your mind with the meaning of the words. Otherwise, there is the danger of your just rushing through the prayers and your mind remaining unmoved by them.

However, as I have already mentioned and as I always explain to Westerners, taking refuge is not simply reciting prayers. You can take verbal refuge, in either English, Tibetan, or Sanskrit, or you can do it silently; the main thing is what is happening in your mind. If you have perfect devotion and continuous understanding that the everlasting, blissful transcendental wisdom is your ultimate goal, with the joy of constantly striving to discover it in your heart, there is no such time that you are not taking refuge. But if you do not have this understanding, even though you say "Namo gurubhya, namo buddhaya..." a million times, nothing happens. It is just a waste of time and energy.

In the Mahayana Buddhist tradition we have the preparatory purifying practices of taking refuge one hundred thousand times, offering one hundred thousand mandalas, doing one hundred thousand prostrations, and so forth. This is to make sure that we do these things not only with our bodies and our speech, but also with our hearts. You can rattle off "Namo buddhaya, namo dharmaya, namo sanghaya" and think that you have finished taking refuge, but it is possible that while your mouth has been taking refuge, your mind has been taking Coca-Cola. Then what benefit have you derived from the words you have been chanting? Perhaps certain words do have some power of their own, but even so, it is questionable that they would have had much effect on you if your mind has been fully occupied by attachment and you have been saying them unconsciously.

Thus, you can see that it is not necessarily easy to take refuge. And when a group of people take refuge together, each person is doing something different. The way one takes refuge depends upon one's understanding and realizations, and these differ from person to person. Even though we all chant the same words or recite the same mantra, each of us feels a unique vibration, which accords to the level and experience of the individual mind.

When you start actualizing bodhicitta, you will find many ways to help other sentient beings. The bodhisattva's duty is to complete the six transcendental perfections, but it takes a long time to gain full realization of these. It is not just one or two days' work. When you practice the perfections, you feel that you are making good use of your life. If you feel that you are not doing anything useful and that you cannot help any sentient being, you are most unwise. Your concern for your problems alone will make you narrower and narrower. You will obsess, "I have so many problems...this problem...that problem...my problem...my problem," and thus remain unaware of the problems faced by mother sentient beings throughout the extent of space. As a result, you will feel no compassion for them.

Such self-obsession causes people to commit suicide. Don't admire them because you think they have finally understood their own problem. People who commit suicide do not understand their problem at all. That's why they kill themselves. Their view is narrow. Suicide is never the result of realizations.

In ancient India there was a king who killed his father. When he realized what he had done he was overcome with remorse, completely depressed, and almost unable to think. Finally, he sought advice from the Buddha, who told him, "Killing your parents is worthwhile." Somehow, he was jolted awake by these words, and his mind started functioning normally again. He thought deeply about what the Buddha had said, and finally realized that what the Buddha was really saying was that he should kill the attachment and deluded mind that give birth to his samsara. Through that realization he became an arhat. The point here is that he became so worried and obsessed by his own problems that these ignorant emotions filled his mind and left no room for understanding wisdom. If our minds get so narrow that we cannot benefit even ourselves, how can we possibly expect to be able to benefit others?

THE VASE MEDITATION: THE NINE-ROUND BREATHING EXERCISE

After you have taken refuge and your objects of refuge have melted into light and dissolved into you, meditate single-pointedly for as long as you can on being one with Heruka or Vajradhara, depending upon which of these deities you visualized as your object of refuge. When dualistic thoughts start to arise, generate bodhicitta, as I explained before.

From this point of the sadhana, you no longer visualize yourself in your ordinary form; instead, you appear in the divine aspect of Heruka or Vajradhara. Thus, you no longer feel, "I am so-and-so..." or imagine that your body is made of flesh, blood, and bone—but neither do you hold the divine pride of being the deity. This means that you visualize yourself as the deity but do not generate the belief that you *are* the deity. Later, you will do the same thing as you recite the purification mantra when practicing the power of the remedy.[6]

Now, while holding the divine appearance of yourself as the deity, you do the vase meditation. In this practice, breathe only though your nose; keep your mouth closed. Inhale and exhale slowly, naturally, and completely, but a little more strongly in the middle of the breath than at the beginning or the end. We say that the pattern of each breath resembles the shape of a barley grain, which is pointed at the ends and wide in the middle. We do not use the forceful method of breathing found in some of the practices of Hindu yoga.

There are many psychic energy channels in your body. Here, we visualize the three main ones. The central channel is a transparent tube in the nature of light about the width of your little finger in diameter running straight down the center of your body from your crown chakra to the chakra at the base of your spine, just in front of your spinal column. The right and left channels are also transparent tubes in the nature of light but are narrower than the central channel. They run from your nostrils up toward the crown chakra, where they curve over like an umbrella handle to run down alongside the central channel, parallel with it, to a point about four fingers' breadth below the level of your navel, where they curve inward and join the central channel.

Having visualized these channels, first breathe in through the left nostril: slowly, then slightly more forcefully, then slowly again. Visualize that the air enters the left channel, filling it completely, and passes down and across into the right channel, up through it and out of the right nostril. This air pushes out all the energy and impressions of your desire and attachment, and these are pushed out beyond the earth's gravitational field, out of this solar system, to disappear forever. Do this three times.

Concentrate fully on the passage of the air through the channels, letting your mind become one with the movement of the air energy. Don't think about what your neighbor is doing or anything else. Do not regard your channels as physical, made of flesh and blood. Remember: you are visualizing yourself in the pure aspect of the deity and the channels are in the nature of consciousness. But since you are not holding the divine pride of being the deity, you can still purify the delusions as I have described.

Repeat the exercise three times, now breathing in through the right nostril and expelling the air through the left. As the air goes down through the right channel and up through the left it pushes out all the energy and impressions of your hatred and aversion—whatever makes you feel dark and uncomfortable. These also pass out of the solar system and vanish into emptiness.

Now breathe in through both nostrils together, bringing the air down through the right and left channels to the point where they join the central channel. To help you concentrate on this you can swallow some saliva as the air goes down. When the air reaches the central channel, tighten the inner pelvic muscles and draw energy up from the lower chakra through the central channel to the navel chakra, where it meets and mixes with the air energy from above. Hold your breath and concentrate on the blissful energy you can feel at this point. This is important. As soon as you no longer feel comfortable, exhale naturally through your nostrils, but visualize that instead of going out, the air you have been holding goes up and dissolves inside the central channel. Do this three times.

This exercise is very helpful for generating blissful energy within your nervous system. The experience of bliss is an integral part of the method of tantric yoga, and thus, this exercise is also helpful for your tantric practice. It is this blissful energy, which is in fact your mind—and it is *your* mind, not somebody else's—that transforms into the lotus seat and the syllable HUM when you go on to practice the rest of the sadhana.

Therefore, make sure that by the end of the vase meditation you feel calm and blissful and that your mind is in no way involved in thoughts of samsaric activities or old familiar places. You should feel that you have such control over your mind that you could place it on any meditation object you choose. If your mind is bothered and agitated, you cannot meditate. Another benefit of this exercise is that it destroys your exaggerated, emotional superstitions, which keep you from accomplishing the yoga method.

Thus, it is important to experience bliss at the navel chakra as you are holding your breath and concentrating there. And simultaneously, you are clearly, consciously aware of that blissful feeling. This is the exact opposite of ordinary samsaric pleasure, which you normally experience unconsciously, without awareness. Why are these two experiences so different? Because one derives from wisdom, the other from ignorance;

one becomes the path of liberation, the other brings more attachment, desire, and conflict into your mind. But through practice, you can discover all this for yourselves; there is no need for me to tell you.

Visualizing the energy dissolving within the central channel when you exhale is an essential aspect of the practice of kundalini yoga. Therefore, it is important to do this and not feel that you are losing the energy at that time. When you have finished the nine rounds of the vase meditation, you can then go on to the actual yoga method.

4

The Actual Yoga Method

The Initial Visualization

Out of the void, about six inches above the crown of my head, appears the seed syllable PAM, which transforms into a thousand-petalled lotus. On top of the lotus appears the seed syllable ah, which transforms into a moon disc. In the center of the moon disc stands the seed syllable HUM. Suddenly, the HUM transforms into a white five-pronged vajra that has a HUM at its center. Much radiant light emanates from both the hum and the vajra, going out into the ten directions and completing the two purposes. The whole universe melts into light. This light then returns to and is absorbed by the HUM in the vajra. The hum and vajra also melt into light and transform into Heruka Vajrasattva.

Vajrasattva is white. He has one face and two arms. He holds a vajra in his right hand and a bell in his left. He is sitting in the full lotus position with his hands in the embracing mudra. His consort, Dorje Nyem-ma, embraces him, her legs encircling his body. She is white and has one face and two arms. She holds a curved knife in her right hand and a skull cup in her left.

They are both dressed in robes of heavenly silk and adorned by precious jewel ornaments. [They both have seed syllables] OM at the crown chakra, AH at the throat chakra, and HUM at the heart. Brilliant light radiates from the HUM at the heart, invoking the divine supreme wisdom energy of all tathagatas.

OUT OF THE SPHERE OF SUNYATA, a few inches above the crown of your head, appears the white syllable PAM, which transforms into a white, thousand-petalled lotus. On the lotus appears a white syllable AH, which transforms into a white moon disc. This moon is nothing like the physical moon that scientists examine, but is in the nature of radiant light. On the moon, at its center, appears a white syllable HUM, which transforms into a white five-pronged vajra, marked at its center by a HUM. The vajra is in the nature of transcendental blissful wisdom.

From the vajra, and especially from the HUM at its center, radiant light shines forth in the ten directions, filling the entire universe. This light accomplishes two purposes. It becomes an offering to all the gurus and buddhas, filling them with a feeling of great blissful energy and joy. The light also reaches all mother sentient beings, purifying their body, speech, and mind of all defilements and negative imprints. All sentient beings and their environments—all animate and inanimate phenomena—melt completely into light, which returns to dissolve into the HUM at the center of the vajra.

The vajra also melts into light, out of which Heruka Vajrasattva suddenly appears. He is white and has one face and two arms. He holds a vajra in his right hand and a bell in his left. He is sitting in the full lotus position with his hands crossed in the embracing mudra.

He embraces his consort Dorje Nyem-ma, who is also white and sits with her legs encircling his hips. She has one face and two arms. She holds a curved knife in her right hand and a nectar-filled skull cup (*kapala)* in her right. The knife symbolizes wisdom; its purpose is to cut wrong conceptions, the ego's projections, and gravitational attachment to sense pleasures. The nectar-filled kapala shows that she has attained the everlasting blissful realization of enlightenment and is not simply an up-and-down worldly woman. Although she is just symbolic, she really gives a great impression.

If you check back through history, you will find that women have usually been considered worthless, nothing but mere servants for men. But they are not. The greatest of Lord Buddha's psychological methods, tantric yoga, shows clearly that women and men are equally capable of discovering the everlasting peaceful transcendental wisdom that lies within the minds of all. Furthermore, women have a special potential to generate the power of wisdom and can thus give great blissful energy to other yogis. At the same time, they receive blissful energy back. Therefore, if you have the inner experience of what the consort symbolizes, every time you see a Mahayana painting, a deep positive imprint is placed upon your mind, and you receive transcendental wisdom. In fact, these paintings are talking to you, beyond words.

Our ignorant, limited mind always thinks, "I can't do anything...I can't do this...I can't do that...," which is completely untrue. You can do whatever you want! Your precious human rebirth offers you so much: you can communicate, think intelligently, and develop yourself infinitely. If you think you are lazy, you will become lazy. You will waste your whole life and will do nothing, simply because you believe that you are incapable of doing anything. You keep pushing yourself down. But this is not true; you are capable of so much!

Tantric yoga shows you the powerful qualities that exist within you and stops you from thinking that you cannot do anything. You are extremely fortunate to have met and understood these teachings and to be putting them into practice. It would be very wise of you to take as much advantage of this opportunity as possible.

If ordinary people saw a painting of Dorje Nyem-ma holding the kapala full of the nectar of blissful energy, symbolizing her attainment of the realization of everlasting joy, they would think that she was some kind of blood-drinking demon. They would be revolted and afraid, thinking that the kapala held human blood and that Mahayana Buddhists believed in human sacrifice. They might even be scared of our cutting their throats! If they saw paintings of Yamantaka wearing human bones, they would feel sick; their superstitions would project that he kills human beings. Contrary to their superstitions, however, these symbols have deep significance and reflect the supreme, highest realizations.

During the sadhana of Heruka Vajrasattva or the six-session guru yoga, there is a part where you have to visualize yourself as Vajrasattva embracing the consort. Now, monks and nuns have vowed not to have sexual contact, and it might be thought that they should not practice this kind of sadhana. However, the consort is not a physical female but a samadhi female, and therefore, it is permitted for monks and nuns to engage in these meditations. Women can visualize themselves either as Vajrasattva embracing the consort or as the consort, Dorje Nyem-ma, herself, who is completely one with Heruka Vajrasattva and his blissful transcendental wisdom. Thus, we transform our negative energy into the blissful transcendental wisdom of Vajrasattva.

The purpose of consort practice is to develop the blissful transcendental wisdom of sunyata. This is the exact opposite of the purpose of the ordinary male-female embrace. In order to be able to embrace with blissful transcendental awareness, it is necessary to gradually develop the mind of blissful transcendental awareness. Therefore, yogis and yoginis first cut any physical contact and practice the yoga method with a samadhi female until they have gained higher realizations. Only when they have reached a higher stage of development can they embrace physically, but it has nothing to do with unconscious samsaric pleasures. There is a long way for us to go to reach that point, and it may not even be necessary for us to do those practices. Therefore, I do not need to give any more details about them now.

Here, the point is that the consort symbolizes helping other yogis to develop everlasting blissful wisdom. If women can do this, it's fine, but if their effect on men is to make them agitated, depressed, discouraged, and unhappy, then everything just becomes samsaric. Naturally, the same can be said about the effect of men upon women.

Both Heruka Vajrasattva and his consort are dressed in garments of heavenly silk and adorned with beautiful jeweled ornaments. Of course, "beautiful" here is relative. What people from one country might find beautiful, people from another might find ugly. According to Buddhist philosophy, beautiful and ugly and good and bad depend on sentient beings' minds. What is ornamental and what is not is all in the mind.

You can understand this simply by looking at the development of Western civilization and how at different times people have considered certain things beautiful and others ugly. You probably understand all this much better than I do. I only know about these things through having studied Buddhist philosophy; you know about them through direct observation of reality. All you have to do is watch how shopkeepers keep changing their displays all the time. What was beautiful yesterday is ugly today, and so it goes. You are lucky! You can see Buddha's philosophy right there, simply by looking at what is going on around you all the time. You don't have to bother so much with technical terms and scriptures. You can enjoy life in your own country and come to understand reality at the same time.

Since people from different countries have their own ideas about what ornaments are beautiful, you might not like the way I describe those adorning Vajrasattva and his consort. Perhaps you'd like to visualize their ornaments in a way more attractive to your tastes. But the ornaments symbolize particular inner realizations and should therefore be visualized as described in the text. Certainly, you should not leave them out just because you think they are too complicated to visualize.

Heruka Vajrasattva has six different kinds of ornament, his consort five. The sixth is a white substance that is applied to his body in a certain way to indicate that he has the kundalini energy realization; it is not smeared all over his body in the way that you might have seen Indian *sadhus* cover themselves with ash. Some men look like men but are impotent; their male energy does not function. This sixth ornament shows that Vajrasattva's kundalini energy is functioning, that he has the kundalini energy realization and can have the experience of transcendental, simultaneously born bliss. (I say "kundalini energy" instead of just "kundalini" so that you will not think that I am referring to the ordinary male energy.)

Both Heruka Vajrasattva and his consort have the syllables OM at the crown chakra, AH at the throat chakra, and HUM at the heart chakra. The HUM is standing at the center of a moon disc. This moon is completely full and symbolizes transcendental great bliss. When you feel hot and go outside to cool off under a full moon, you automatically feel cool and happy. This is one of the reasons that a full moon has been chosen to symbolize great bliss. Around the edge of the moon disc stand the syllables of the Heruka Vajrasattva mantra, reading counterclockwise. Usually in tantric sadhanas, the mantra reads clockwise—from left to right; here, it reads counterclockwise, from right to left, to show that Heruka Vajrasattva emphasizes female energy more than male. It is said that women use the energy of the left side of their body more than the right, while men use the right more than the left.

When Buddhists circumambulate a stupa, they usually walk clockwise, keeping the stupa to their right. As a practitioner of female tantra, conscious of what you are doing, you could go around in the opposite direction. People who don't have a higher understanding might just think you are wrong, and simply trying to be different; those who do understand might be very impressed by your obvious knowledge of secret mantra. However, it is not good to show off, and you should just try to be simple and act conventionally.

From the HUM at the divine heart of Heruka Vajrasattva, much radiant light goes out in all directions, invoking the supreme pure energy of the wisdom of all buddhas, which returns in the form of light to dissolve back into the HUM.

MAKING OFFERINGS TO HERUKA VAJRASATTVA

OM KHANDA ROHI HUM HUM PHAT
OM SVABHAVA SHUDDAH SARVA DHARMA SVABHAVA SHUDDHO HAM

All is void. A seed syllable AH appears out of the void. It turns into a huge white kapala containing the five meats and the five nectars. They melt, becoming an ocean of the amrita-energy of divine transcendental wisdom.

OM AH HUM HA HO HRI

Next you recite the mantra to purify and bless the offerings and make their energy inexhaustible (OM KHANDA...). It is similar to making the inner offering. You are in the aspect of Heruka Vajrasattva, and you bless the offerings.

Then recite the sunyata mantra (OM SVABHAVA...). All becomes empty. With the sunyata mantra and the right view of emptiness, you transform the offerings and all other phenomena in the universe into blissful transcendental wisdom. Out of non-duality appears the white syllable AH, which turns into a huge white kapala. Inside this there are the five kinds of meat and the five nectars. They melt, blend, and become a vast ocean of nectar, the essence of which is blissful divine wisdom.

Then recite the mantra OM AH HUM HA HO HRI three times. Here, we purify the impure energy of the offering ingredients, removing faults of taste, smell, color, and power, or potential; we transform it into nectar; and we increase it, making it inexhaustible.

I am sure that many of you could have some kind of sunyata experience in meditation, but the trouble is that whenever you perceive a sense object your dualistic mind automatically grasps at it, and you fall back into your old habitual samsaric mind patterns. It is completely different if you have blissful divine wisdom. No matter what you perceive, your mind does not move, grasp, or cling; you have complete, joyful freedom. You see the absolute nature of all phenomena in the universe and experience everything with bliss.

OM VAJRASATTVA ARGHAM...SHABDA PRATICCHA HUM SVAHA

Thus, we make the eight offerings to Heruka Vajrasattva. One needs transcendental wisdom to make them perfectly; we should at least have deep understanding and intelligence.

Ordinary tourists who see altars in Tibetan temples and monasteries judge everything by external appearances and worldly modes of thought. They really believe that we offer food, paper, water, and cloth to graven images and other physical objects. They even get upset by some of the statues, such as those of wrathful deities grasping human beings between their fangs, and cannot believe how the stupid heathens could possibly make offerings to such hideous figures. Be careful: if your wisdom is a little weak you too could think like this.

However, making material offerings is a highly beneficial practice. It stops you from being lazy and hypocritical, rationalizing, "Oh, I make offerings mentally," and never reaching into your pocket to give even a few cents. I'm sure you know what I mean. But if you offer only one candle with correct understanding and the proper visualization, it is as if you were offering the entire universe and everything in it. Also, most of us have small minds and cannot visualize. It is difficult for us mentally to offer the entire universe. The eight material offerings make it easier by serving as a base that we can transform into everything magnificent in the universe.

You should not see any offering as an ordinary, samsaric object of enjoyment; instead, transform it into blissful transcendental wisdom that then manifests as nectar-like water, light, sound, taste, smell, and touch. Through this practice you can realize that anything on earth, whatever its outer form, is a transformation of blissful transcendental wisdom. Western science has already shown that all energy is in a constant state of flux; one form of energy is always changing into another. For example, the energy of the sun interacts with that of a plant, and a beautiful flower emerges. Everything in the world is capable of change.

Whenever you visualize blissful transcendental wisdom in any of its aspects, your mind reflects it automatically; all the negative, foggy, obstructive energy of your wrong conceptions is displaced by wisdom. Joyful energy arises spontaneously in your mind, without your having to depend on chocolate and cake! If you experiment, you will easily discover how this exceptional psychology works.

Many people want to kill themselves. Their problem is their visualization. All they can see is suffering and conflict; they cannot forget their worries, they cannot sleep. Suicide is their only solution; they slash their wrists. It is important that you understand the psychology of suicide.

It is just as important that you understand the psychology and the real purpose of making offerings. If you do not understand the transcendental nature of the materials you offer, they remain physical objects, and your offering is an empty ritual. But if you understand their nature, you can see how making offerings is a profound and perfect treatment for the deluded mind: peaceful, gentle, and full of wisdom. If you train yourself in this kind of visualization, you will never have a depressed or pessimistic view of the world.

Do not look down on the practice of transformation. A drink turned into blissful nectar tastes far better than any drink samsara can offer. Even the best tea or coffee gives you only a little bit of pleasure between your mouth and your stomach. Its energy is fleeting, and soon after drinking it you have to go to the toilet. Divine nectar, on the other hand, dissolves into your entire nervous system, giving bliss to all five senses, and the energy you get from it is beyond compare. Really! I am not exaggerating.

Some people think that monks and nuns have to renounce music. We renounce nothing! We enjoy and offer every beautiful sound in the universe. We do not miss out on singing and dancing either. We can sing and dance as much as we like, as long as we remain in single-pointed concentration, conscious and liberated, and do not shake or upset our nervous systems. In Tibetan monasteries and nunneries they play musical instruments in pujas and do religious dances, too. We don't miss out on life, we gain from it!

Of course, if you try to explain all this to Westerners, they will think you are either crazy or dreaming. But it is neither madness nor a dream; it is reality. If they disagree,ask them, "What, then, is reality?" They cannot answer. They think they are very intelligent; that what they are doing is reality, while what we are doing is a fantasy. This is a wrong conception. If you analyze with skillful wisdom, you will find that basically we are both doing the same thing—they're hallucinating; we're hallucinating. So what's true for one is true for the other.

The offerings you make have three characteristics: their essence is blissful transcendental wisdom; this wisdom manifests as the various objects of offering; and each object gives its own kind of inexhaustible, everlasting pleasure to the senses.

You can visualize that the eight offerings are being made by eight goddesses. When you snap your fingers at the beginning of each offering mudra, the appropriate goddess emanates from your heart and makes the offering, after which she dissolves back into your heart as you finish the mudra with a second snap of your fingers. The goddesses are manifestations of divine transcendental wisdom; when they dissolve into you, their immaculate purity and beauty brings indescribable bliss into your heart. Each has four arms: their first right and left hands hold a vajra and bell; their other two hold the appropriate offering.

The eight offerings and their goddesses are:

argham	Nectar Goddess	(*Chö-yön-ma*), white in color
padyam	Foot-bathing Goddess	(*Zhab-sil-ma*), white
pushpe	Flower Goddess	(*Me-tog-ma*), white
dhupe	Incense Goddess	(*Dug-pö-ma*), smoke-colored
aloke	Light Goddess	(*Nang-säl-ma*), red
gandhe	Perfume Goddess	(*Dri-chab-ma*), green
naivedya	Food Goddess	(*Zhäl-sä-ma*), multi-colored
shabda	Sound Goddess	(*Dra-chog-ma*), blue

JAH HUM BAM HO. [The wisdom beings] become non-dual [with the symbolic beings].

Having made the offerings, we recite the mantra JAH HUM BAM HO. With JAH, the divine wisdom is invoked; with HUM, the divine wisdom enters; with BAM, it becomes non-dual unity; and with HO, it becomes blissfully indestructible.

Thus, the energy of the divine wisdom of all buddhas that we invoked before is magnetically attracted by the light that radiates from the HUM at the heart of Heruka Vajrasattva. Instantaneously and effortlessly, it dissolves into his heart, becoming blissfully one with his divine wisdom, like a drop of water merging with the ocean, no longer separate or dual.

Actually, Heruka Vajrasattva has no need to invoke divine wisdom; he is already one with all buddhas. It is quite wrong to think that Heruka Vajrasattva is one thing and that all buddhas are something else. But the problem is that your dualistic mind does not understand that the divine form you are visualizing above the crown of your head and the divine wisdom from which it manifests are perfectly one. You instinctively distinguish them as separate. Therefore, you need to trick your dualistic mind with this kind of visualization.

Also, it is no good simply saying, "Oh yes, they are one and the same," if your knowledge is merely intellectual. This does not help your mind develop. However, when you experience the real meaning of oneness through your practice of the yoga method, your realization of it becomes entirely intuitive. Heruka Vajrasattva is the combined pure energy of all buddhas manifesting in that divine aspect to communicate with you. When you have fully purified your dualistic mind, you too will be one with this blissful transcendental wisdom.

THE INITIATION

Again, brilliant light radiates from the hum at the divine heart, invoking all initiating deities of the five families.

OM PANCHA KULA SAPARIVARA ARGHAM...SHABDA PRATICCHA HUM SVAHA

"All tathagatas, please bestow on me the [Heruka Vajrasattva] initiation." Upon this request, all the tathagatas hold up their initiation vases, which are full of the amrita energy of divine transcendental wisdom, and the amrita starts to flow. As the mantra OM SARVA TATHAGATA ABHISHEKATA SAMAYA SHRIYE HUM *is said, the initiation is conferred.*

The divine body of perfect absolute wisdom, Heruka Vajrasattva, is completely filled by the amrita energy of blissful transcendental wisdom. Some amrita overflows and turns into Akshobhya, who adorns his crown.

The seed syllable HUM *stands at the center of a moon disc at the divine heart, encircled by the one hundred syllable mantra [standing counterclockwise around the edge of the moon disc].*

Once again, much light radiates from the HUM at the divine heart of Heruka Vajrasattva, filling all of space in the ten directions and invoking the principal initiators—the five *dhyani* buddhas—and all other buddhas, in their tantric aspects, for the initiation. Again, magnetically attracted by the light, they come in an instant into the space above and around Heruka Vajrasattva's head.

Now, before requesting these buddhas for the initiation, make them the same eight offerings as above. When you say PRATICCHA HUM SVAHA you are asking them please to accept each of these offerings, whose nature is divine wisdom, and experience the joy of blissful transcendental wisdom in their holy minds.

Having made the offerings, you request the initiation. As you recite the mantra OM SARVA TATHAGATA..., the initiators then grant your request, conferring the initiation by lifting up the initiation vases and pouring the purifying nectar of divine transcendental wisdom into the central channels of Heruka Vajrasattva and Dorje Nyem-ma through their crown chakras.

It looks to you as if you are down here visualizing Heruka Vajrasattva up there, taking the initiation on your behalf. Again, this is because of your dualistic imprints of, "I am this, he is that." To destroy the ordinary conceptions and projections of the dualistic mind, you need purifying visualizations such as this.

The whole point of this yoga method is to purify your own mind. Although you visualize Heruka Vajrasattva being purified, psychologically you are purifying yourself. Your visualization of Heruka Vajrasattva is your own impure vision. By purifying him with the most profound, pure, clean-clear energy of enlightenment, you yourself become pure. This leaves a deep imprint on your consciousness and automatically releases you from negative energy.

After the initiation, the divine body of Heruka Vajrasattva is completely full of the energy of the nectar of blissful transcendental wisdom that the initiating buddhas have poured through his crown chakra into his central channel. If you have the great wisdom of tantric yoga, you can have the same experience yourself.

You should realize, however, that your entire nervous system is, in fact, *already* full of the energy of blissful nectar. But instead, you always think you are poor, that something is always missing from your life: "I don't have this, I don't have that, I don't have the other." Then you think, "If only I had this, I'd be happy." You are constantly dissatisfied and always looking for whatever it is that you think you do not have.

Your lower chakra is dark, blocked, painful, and devoid of blissful energy. Your naval chakra is dark, depressed, and closed. Your broken heart chakra is drowning in the blood of emotions of hopelessness. Your throat chakra is completely defiled, and nothing you say is positive. And your frozen head chakra is as hard, cold, and inflexible as an igloo, unmelted by the fire within. You are too impure, and give blissful energy to neither yourself nor others. Everything is dark, blocked, and defiled.

However, through this yoga method you can realize the greatest wisdom and bring its everlasting blissful energy into your innermost heart. You can use the techniques of this highest yoga method from now until you die. Even after death we can use them, because we are constantly developing. If we do not develop, our minds will always be up and down, dualistic, and we shall never be happy. Look at how we are: we have studied so much Dharma but still we are running around doing this and that. Samsaric activities are endless. Even those of us who live in monasteries and meditation centers, which are supposed to be places of peace and quiet that everybody likes, are busy, busy, busy. Life is sure to finish soon, that's all.

In the sadhana there is the Tibetan word *ku; kaya* in Sanskrit. We translate this term into English as "divine body" or "holy body," but perhaps "pure nervous system" would be better. I don't know what the right scientific term should be to translate these Tibetan and Sanskrit words, but I'm sure that we have all had some experience of what these words connote. *Ku* implies that the pure nervous system of Heruka Vajrasattva is pervaded by everlasting blissful kundalini energy.

Our nervous systems are pervaded by this blissful energy too, but we don't recognize it. However, we have all had feelings of joy in our minds and physical nervous systems, when our negative energy has transformed into bliss and we have not clung to any external object, and have been able to maintain control. But despite such experiences we continue to act under the influence of the old imprints of our wrong conceptions. Of course, I know these conceptions are strong, but we should try to overcome them as hard as we can, according to our understanding of these pure blissful experiences. It is simply a question of taking advantage of the opportunities offered us. We should learn from our small experiences of bliss.

For example, if someone were to ask you to choose between lunch at a beautiful five-star hotel and chapatis in a dirty Indian tea shop, you would not hesitate to choose the big hotel. In the same way, here we have the chance to experience within our nervous systems the everlasting bliss of the internal five-star lunch, but we still choose the dirty chapati. Why? Because of our grasping emotional attitude and wrong conceptions. This shows clearly how ignorant and neurotic we really are. Check up, you'll see!

Now not only does the nectar completely fill Heruka Vajrasattva's pure nervous system, but it also overflows, the excess nectar turning into the *dhyani buddha* Akshobhya, who adorns the crown of Vajrasattva's head. There are different ways of interpreting the significance of this, but here it shows that Heruka Vajrasattva is in the energy stream of the buddha Akshobhya. You will remember that during an initiation there is a part where you discover to which of the five dhyani buddhas you are most closely connected, and after that, you are supposed to maintain your contact with that buddha's energy stream. This visualization relates to that.

Having given the initiation, all the buddhas melt into the divine heart of Heruka Vajrasattva, their blissful transcendental wisdom becoming inseparably one with his. Again, this visualization of the initiating buddhas not returning to their original places but dissolving into Vajrasattva's heart has profound psychological significance and benefit in terms of your developing the realization of union-oneness.

At the center of a moon disc at Heruka Vajrasattva's divine heart stands the seed syllable HUM, surrounded by the letters of the hundred syllable Heruka Vajrasattva mantra standing counterclockwise around the edge of the moon disc.

OFFERINGS AND PRAISE TO HERUKA VAJRASATTVA

OM VAJRASATTVA ARGHAM...SHABDA PRATICCHA HUM SVAHA
OM VAJRASATTVA OM AH HUM

Non-dual divine wisdom, magnificent inner jewel ornament of all mother sentient beings; supreme, unchanging, everlasting great bliss; indestructible, magnificent wisdom mind that releases all sentient beings from all negativities of body, speech, and mind, especially broken vows and pledges: to you I prostrate.

(Optional: long or short outer mandala offerings.)

SECRET MANDALA

The right view of sunyata is one with the wisdom of great bliss. This wisdom transforms into Mount Meru, the sun, the moon, and all other phenomena in the universe. I offer everything magnificent to you, ocean of great kindness, the one who is liberated and who liberates all others as well.

INNER MANDALA

Please bless me and all other sentient beings to be released immediately from the three poisons, for I am offering without the slightest hesitation or attachment all objects of my greed, hatred, and ignorance; friends, enemies, and strangers; and my body and all possessions. Please accept all this.

Make the eight offerings as you did before. These are followed by the inner offering (Tib. *nang-chö*).

Our samsaric mind views all phenomena as either pure or impure, and dualistically we grasp at and cling to the objects that constitute our impermanent five aggregates. Through the yoga method we transform our five aggregates into blissful transcendental wisdom, which is beyond duality and of the nature of the five dhyani buddhas, and offer it. That is why it is called the inner offering.

Next, we praise the divine wisdom of non-duality, the magnificent inner jewel ornament of all mother sentient beings, whose nature is unchanging, everlasting great bliss. This is Heruka Vajrasattva, who by the power of that blissful wisdom releases all mother sentient beings from all the negative energy of broken vows and non-virtuous actions of body, speech, and mind. We prostrate to that sublime indestructible mind of wisdom.

Then we offer the mandala. In the secret mandala offering we are saying that the understanding of the ultimate nature, sunyata, is one with blissful, simultaneously born wisdom. This wisdom is transformed into Mount Meru, the sun and the moon, and all other phenomena in the universe. We offer the magnificence of all existence to Heruka Vajrasattva, the ocean of great kindness who is himself liberated and who liberates all others as well.

5

The Purification

"Bhagawan Vajrasattva, please purify all negativities and broken and damaged pledges of myself and other sentient beings."

Because of this request, brilliant light radiates from the mantra rosary and the HUM *at the divine heart. It purifies all negativities and obscurations of all sentient beings and becomes an offering for all buddhas and bodhisattvas. The essence of the perfect qualities of their holy body, speech, and mind returns in the form of light, which dissolves into the* HUM *and the mantra rosary.*

[From the HUM *and the mantra rosary] a stream of blissful white amrita energy begins to flow down through the chakras of the divine couple. It flows out through the chakra of union and enters my crown chakra. This stream of amrita of transcendental wisdom fills my whole body, destroying all the negativities and obscurations of my body, speech, and mind. These are completely purified.*

FIRST YOU REQUEST Heruka Vajrasattva—destroyer of all defilements, who possesses all realizations and has transcended this world—to purify you and all other sentient beings of all negativities of body, speech, and mind and all broken and degenerated tantric pledges and commitments.

Much light radiates from the HUM and mantra rosary at the divine hearts of Heruka Vajrasattva and his consort, filling all of space in the ten directions, purifying the negativities of all sentient beings and making offerings for the enjoyment of the buddhas and their sons, the bodhisattvas. The pure essence of the transcendental wisdom of all holy beings' body, speech, and mind returns in the form of light, dissolving into the HUM and mantra rosary at the hearts of Vajrasattva and his consort. From these, vast quantities of blissful white kundalini (*amrita*) energy pour down his central channel. The essence of this kundalini energy is his blissful transcendent wisdom. Its energy is inexhaustible—the exact opposite of our limited energy, which always runs out quickly and requires us to eat to replenish it. When you are doing this visualization, you should also visualize the blissful white kundalini energy pouring down the central channel of Heruka Vajrasattva's consort, Dorje Nyem-ma.

The blissful white kundalini energy pours down their central channels, past their navel and sex chakras, and leaves their pure bodies from the point where they are joined in union. It continues down through the moon and lotus seats, which, being in the nature of transcendent wisdom, offer no resistance. It enters you through the crown chakra, rushing down through your central channel with the force of a powerful waterfall. It is very important that you visualize this torrent of white nectar as overwhelmingly powerful. It surges into your body and spreads through your entire system. This white energy is not physical, but somehow it feels incredibly real. You are also filled with radiant light and almost totally overcome with bliss. All defilements of your body, speech, and mind disappear without a trace.

MANTRA RECITATION[7]

OM VAJRA HERUKA SAMAYAM ANUPALAYA. HERUKA TENOPATISHTHA. DRIDHO ME BHAVA, SUTOSHYO ME BHAVA, SUPOSHYO ME BHAVA, ANURAKTO ME BHAVA. SARVA SIDDHIM ME PRAYACCHA. SARVA KARMA SUCHA ME CHITTAM SHREYAH KURU, HUM! HA HA HA HA HOH! BHAGAVAN VAJRA HERUKA MA ME MUNCHA. HERUKA BHAVA MAHA SAMAYA SATTVA AH HUM PHAT!

Now recite the hundred syllable mantra of Heruka Vajrasattva. There are three different meditation techniques for you to use while you recite it. The first is called *yän-de.* The blissful white kundalini energy rushes into your central channel. It spreads throughout your nervous system, flushing out all negativities through the openings and pores of the lower part of your body. There are various ways of visualizing the negativities as they leave your body; you can choose that which is most effective for your mind. You can visualize the three poisonous minds of ignorance, attachment, and aversion coming out in the form of pigs, chickens, and snakes, respectively. Or you can simply visualize all your negative energy in the form of what you consider to be the worst kind of sentient being, such as scorpions, crabs, snakes, and worms, or as thick black tar or dirty sump oil.

Some people might think it strange to be flushing insects, reptiles, and crustaceans from their bodies, but in fact, there are many sentient beings living inside us. We have a symbiotic relationship with some of these and would not survive without them.

Our bodies also harbor worms: long worms, short worms, and many other kinds as well. It is not through chance but through karma that they are there. We are repaying them our karmic debt. In the past we took from them; now they are taking from us. We took their food and left them none; therefore, they have come into our stomach to eat ours. Even the greediest people in the world, who through great attachment cannot share anything with others, have no choice but to share their food when the worms move in. Karma is strong; there is no way out. Even when you get rid of the worms, they return. They take your health and, sometimes, even your life. There are many ways you can lose your life; don't think it needs someone to attack you with a knife or something like that.

Feel that you have been completely purified, especially of gross negativities. We often say that our old habits are difficult to get rid of, but that's not true; at least, the reasons are not physical—it is our minds that make things difficult. We always feel bliss physically; we are so physically oriented. We believe things to be physically difficult for all sorts of external reasons. When things aren't going well we blame our parents: "My mother did this; my father did that. My mother is like this; my father like that...." It is not our bodies but our minds that make life difficult.

If it really were your body alone that caused problems, how could you sit cross-legged for as long as you do? You were not brought up to sit like that. It is your mind that allows you to do so. When you sit cross-legged and meditate, you feel comfortable, your mind is more easily controlled, and that small experience gives you enough interest to continue. As you do so, you feel increasingly comfortable. This does not come about for physical reasons; such control comes from your mind. Therefore, the process of the yoga method is for the blissful transcendental energy to wash away your ego and gravitational attachment to sense pleasures, leaving you completely purified.

The next technique to use while reciting the mantra is called *män-de.* Here, the blissful kundalini energy fills your entire nervous system, starting at the bottom and going all the way up to the top. As it rises, all your negativities float up on the surface of this blissful energy and exit through the openings and pores of the upper part of your body. It is similar to the way that garbage lying at the bottom of a bucket rises to the top as you fill it with water. As the nectar fills your body, you experience great bliss. Feel that you have been completely purified, especially of subtle negativities.

The third visualization is called *phung-de*. Here, the emphasis is on light instead of the white kundalini energy. Limitless blissful radiant light emanates from Heruka Vajrasattva's heart in a powerful beam that bursts through his sex chakra and your crown chakra and enters your central channel. It is white but has a rainbow-like quality with red, yellow, green, and blue in it as well. The instant this brilliant light enters your body it completely dispels the darkness of your doubt-wracked, indecisive mind and your ignorance, attachment, and aversion; all of these disappear forever. It is like switching on a light in a dark room, where the darkness vanishes instantly and no longer exists anywhere. It doesn't go out the window, does it? It simply vanishes. Thus, there is no space for darkness or impurity anywhere in your brain, throat, or any other part of your nervous system. You are as clear as crystal. Feel that you have been completely purified, especially of the most subtle negativities.

When you are in retreat, you can do each of these purifying techniques in each session by dividing the period for mantra recitation into three, or spend an entire session on each method separately, using the next technique in the following session.

When you are not in retreat, it is highly beneficial for you to practice this meditation every day, reciting the Heruka Vajrasattva mantra twenty-one times with each of the three techniques. The best time to do it is at night, just before you go to bed. During the day you are so busy that you are likely to meditate distractedly. Therefore, as the last thing at night, you completely purify all the non-virtues you created during the day and go to sleep feeling free and liberated instead of sad and bothered by the day's negativities. Because we are constantly involved in so much activity, we need a powerful yoga method such as this. There is so little time to purify.

The weight of unpurified negative karmic imprints increases exponentially, but if we recite the Vajrasattva mantra just twenty-one times at the end of each day, even the negative karma of tantric vows broken that day will not increase. If this method has the power to prevent from increasing the negative karma that results from broken tantric root vows—which are the highest vows and most serious transgressions of all—of course it can stop the increase of negativities from actions that are non-virtuous by nature (natural negativities), such as killing and so forth, and other broken vows. Moreover, if we recite this mantra properly one hundred thousand times, all negativities whatsoever can be completely purified.

While you recite the mantra, it is essential that you remain in single-pointed concentration; do not allow any samsaric thoughts to interrupt your meditation. If you can do your practice with good concentration and stable penetrative insight, it will be tremendously effective in eradicating impure concepts and the darkness of emotional obstacles. That purification comes from the power of your concentrated meditation, but the mantra too has power of its own. Sometimes it brings you telepathic visions of things that are happening on the other side of the planet. When you purify the obstacles of narrow emotional concepts, you will discover a whole new world.

Mantra can also enable you to read the minds of others. That can cause you pleasure or pain; it depends what the other person is thinking! Many other things can happen too—it all depends upon the individual; when people retreat, they have different experiences and receive different realizations. It is very difficult for us to tell who has realized what. Some become American Vajrasattvas, some Asian Vajrasattvas, some European Vajrasattvas, some Australian Vajrasattvas...who knows!

6

THE CONCLUDING PRACTICES

OM VAJRASATTVA ARGHAM...SHABDA PRATICCHA HUM SVAHA
OM VAJRASATTVA OM AH HUM

Non-dual divine wisdom...to you I prostrate.

Through ignorance and delusion, I have broken and damaged my pledges. Holy Guru, who has the power to liberate me, my inner master, holder of the vajra, whose essence is great compassion, Lord of all migratory beings, to you I go for refuge.

Vajrasattva says, "Oh son (or daughter) of good family, your negativities and obscurations and damaged and broken pledges are cleansed and purified." Then he dissolves into me. My three doors (of body, speech, and mind) become inseparably one with Vajrasattva's holy body, speech, and mind.

FOLLOWING THE RECITATION of the mantra we again make the eight outer offerings and the inner offering, offer praise to Heruka Vajrasattva as before, and make the prayer of supplication.

You declare to Heruka Vajrasattva that because of unawareness caused by ignorance, you have not known what you have been doing and have acted contrary to the pure energy of your *samaya,* your sacred pledge. Actually, while you are living at a monastery or a meditation center, you can't really assess the progress you have made. It's when you get back home or into the city that your reality shows. While you are practicing in a group, you feel very strong and think that it will be easy to maintain a daily practice, get up for meditation early in the morning, and so forth.

But when you're back home, you sleep late, get up slowly, talk, plan the day with your friends, have breakfast...and all of a sudden it is nine o'clock, and there is no time for meditation because you have to rush off to work. Then, it is lunchtime, teatime, dinnertime, and finally—too late for meditation—bedtime. And so your life finishes. What you really want is wisdom, but you are not doing anything to get it. You spend all your time working for money. You don't give wisdom a chance. Analyze your day and you will see how ridiculously samsaric your life is.

It is not that you really want to destroy yourself; you are not so ignorant that you want to miss out on the blissful energy of transcendental wisdom. But you make your outer world so interesting that you have to spend your whole time watching it. Thus, you never give yourself a chance to sit and meditate on your internal world. The outer world runs day and night; it will rotate forever. And although you don't want it to, your Dharma wisdom declines.

This is like what happens at our Kopan Monastery in Nepal. In the monsoon it rains so much that there is too much water. Then, the sun shines and gradually the water dries up until we are left with dust blowing in the wind. Your Dharma wisdom is like this water: it evaporates until all that is left in your mind is the dust of the defilements. You wonder, "I really thought I had something but there's nothing there. What went wrong?" You feel empty inside. There is wisdom there, but you are not giving it a chance. Wisdom cannot come in a day. First you have to cut your old conceptions, and then slowly, slowly, the vibration of wisdom will grow to guide you.

When students who have lived and studied Dharma in the East go home to the West, that is what happens. Whatever wisdom they have gained decreases without their even noticing. They cannot understand how it happened and can hardly believe that it has. Then, they rationalize, "Oh, what I learned from the lamas must be an Eastern thing. It doesn't work in the West." What doesn't work? If you don't use something, how can it work? If you use Lord Buddha's wisdom, it works; if you don't use it, it doesn't work. It gets rusty! Also, it is very difficult to detect small increases and decreases in wisdom; you have to be very sensitive and watch carefully. Then, you will notice how your mind goes up and down.

If you are not sensitive, if you do not observe your mind, you will never notice what it is doing. This is how dogs behave. A dog's mind is up and down a thousand times a day, but in the evening there is no way for him to analyze his day's experiences. He cannot remember. A dog has no idea whether his mind is developing or degenerating, and neither do you. You should not be like that. While you are preoccupied with your ego's illusory projections, your life is running out.

In the second half of the prayer of supplication you take refuge in your lama, who has the power to liberate other beings. Indians and Nepalis use the word "lama" to refer to any Tibetan. Here it has its true meaning of spiritual master, or guru. He holds in his mind the inner vajra of the great blissful transcendental wisdom, his nature is great kindness and compassion, and he is the leader of all sentient beings.

Then Heruka Vajrasattva replies to you, saying, "My son (or daughter), all your negativities, obscurations, and broken samayas have been completely purified." After that, Dorje Nyem-ma melts into light and dissolves into his heart. Heruka Vajrasattva also melts into light, which enters your central channel and dissolves into your heart. Your three doors of body, speech, and mind and the holy body, speech, and mind of Heruka Vajrasattva become inseparably one. You remain in union-oneness, enjoying the bliss of the sunyata experience with full single-pointed concentration, completely beyond all dualistic views that differentiate between subject and object. This is the highest possible enjoyment.

While you are saying the prayer, you should meditate. After you have finished the prayer, continue meditating with single-pointed concentration on the feeling of unity and avoid all dualistic thoughts of *that-this* and "I am...." You might have noticed that in pujas, Tibetan monks chant and stop, chant and stop. Some people probably think it's weird, but they are meditating on the important points of the practice, not just rushing through it without pausing to think. When you practice the sadhana of Heruka Vajrasattva, you should also do it in this way. And after the dedication, you should not jump up immediately and rush out of the room, but remain a while in single-pointed concentration on your oneness with Heruka Vajrasattva, who is also completely one with your guru.

Make sure that you understand the divine wisdom of Heruka Vajrasattva's holy body, speech, and mind, without projecting, "I am." And also, as I emphasized before, don't have expectations, such as, "Oh, maybe today I'll see Heruka Vajrasattva." Not only is this unnecessary, but it also helps develop your superstitions. So, abandon such thoughts. Also, especially in retreat, don't worry that you're going to get sick. The worry itself will make you sick. Just relax, and have great faith in Guru Heruka Vajrasattva and karma.

DEDICATION

Because of this merit, may I quickly become Heruka Vajrasattva and lead each and every sentient being into his divine enlightened realm.

Part 2

Retreat Instructions

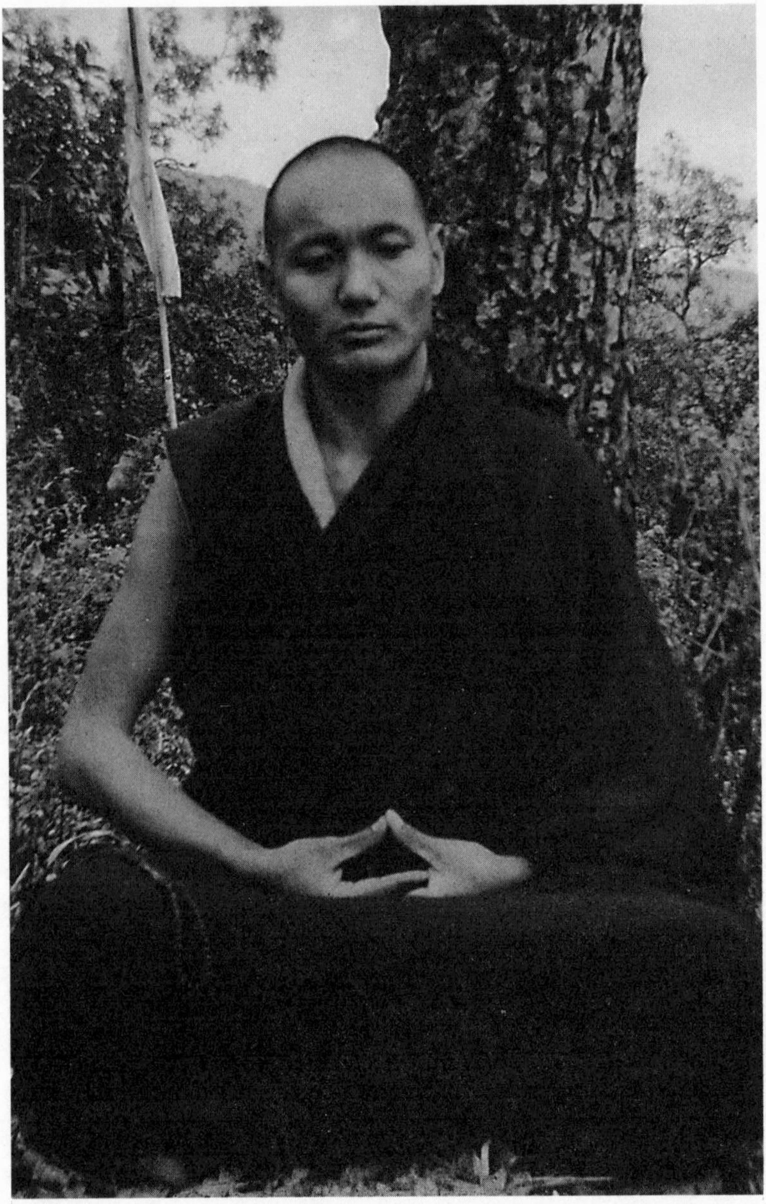

Photograph courtesy of Sister Max Mathews

7

Getting Ready for Retreat

Qualifications for Retreat

What qualifications does a person need in order to retreat on the maha-anuttara yoga tantra aspect of Vajrasattva? The basic requirement is that you be a serious, sincere practitioner, enthusiastically determined to attain the everlasting peaceful realization of enlightenment, and not a hypocrite. Also, you should be practicing what your teacher has shown you—not some misinterpretation projected by your own wrong-conception mind.

The experience of yogis and yoginis in the Tibetan tradition is that, as a general qualification, you must have received teachings on the graduated path to enlightenment in a perfect manner and have been putting them into practice. As the specific qualification, you must have received initiation into the maha-anuttara yoga tantra aspect of Vajrasattva. If you are so qualified, it is possible for you to actualize this practice.

The reason that knowledge and experience of the graduated path to enlightenment is essential is that its three principal aspects—renunciation, bodhicitta, and correct understanding of sunyata—are indispensable prerequisites for the attainment of tantric realizations. Without them, your practice of the yoga method will not be effective. It will remain superficial and intellectual and will never become one with your mind. If on this basis you receive the necessary initiation from a perfectly qualified master, you are fully equipped to make a successful retreat on Heruka Vajrasattva, and most fortunate to be able to do so.

Where to Retreat

Where should a properly qualified person retreat? Will any place do? No—it should be a place that gives you a feeling of reality, not one that is a big hallucination, a polluted projection of the deluded mind.

Sometimes we are not so wise; we try to meditate in a place that's like a furnace and complain when we can't take it any longer. If you stick you finger into a fire, it'll get burnt. You can't then get upset, "My finger's burning!" A fire's nature is to burn. It's up to you to choose the appropriate mandala for the way in which you want to develop…just like you choose shoes that fit your feet!

Of course, if you have great mind control, you can go anywhere; your controlled vibration will even affect others. But if you are weak, the uncontrolled vibration of those around you affects you; even your small candlelight of wisdom will be blown out, and you will finish up in a samsaric supermarket situation. In retreat, we are, in fact, trying to gain control over our minds—but we are babies with a long way to go, when it comes to that. Baby minds need ideal conditions.

In the lamas' experience, the ideal place is a beautiful, natural environment where the atmosphere is quiet, peaceful, and relaxed, where you can see snowy mountains and there are wild flowers, medicinal plants, pleasing, natural smells, and fresh, clean water. You should avoid places that are dirty, close to roads, traffic, and people, or dangerous, or where poisonous plants grow. You should not retreat in a place where you automatically feel insecure and nervous.

Places where holy beings live are excellent: they have a good vibration that I am sure Westerners, who are very sensitive, can feel. Such ideal places are usually very isolated. In Tibet, we used to study in the monasteries and qualify for retreats as explained above, and then go to an isolated place to meditate. These places were extremely simple, not like the Western luxury "retreats" to which rich people escape when they do not want to meet anybody. Westerners really know how to enjoy themselves, even in isolation! However, it is all done out of self-cherishing. Ascetics' retreats are exactly the opposite.

You can also retreat in a monastery or at a Dharma center. In the East, many meditators used to retreat near cemeteries. Such places are usually quiet. You build your hut some distance away from the part of the cemetery that people come to and, with deep understanding of impermanence and death, retreat. The place where you retreat is very important.

A proper retreat place is not necessarily important for everybody, but it is for us. Our minds are like those of babies: easily influenced by external conditions. Actually, our minds are worse than those of babies. Babies grasp at whatever they see, but not only do we grasp at things we see, we intellectualize as well. Also, our wisdom is limited. Therefore, we must put ourselves into the right environment. If our minds were free from confusion, we would have no need to worry about the environment; we wouldn't even need to retreat on Vajrasattva.

It is very important to think carefully about the place in which you are putting yourself—not only where you are going to retreat, but also where you are going to live. Decide what you want to learn, and live near where you can be taught. In Western cities you can choose your environment quite easily. If you want to spend your time at the movies, you can live near a cinema. You have the freedom to do that. In other words, you have some control over your karma, the way your life develops. You cannot say that you are powerless to choose anything because it all depends upon your karma. You create your karma. Your environment depends upon your karma, and you have the ability to direct it. For example, if you want to retreat, you arrange the circumstances so that you can do so. That is creating karma. The result is that you get the chance to retreat and develop your wisdom.

The conclusion is that you have to choose your retreat place very carefully. The best place is one in which you feel secure in the knowledge that from beginning to end, there will be no distractions. Of course, there is no real security in our insecure samsaric lives, but somehow you should feel that the place you have chosen is as good as it is possible to find, and that you will be able to retreat there effectively.

WHEN TO START RETREAT

Generally, the type and purpose of a retreat determine its starting time. Since Heruka Vajrasattva is a mother tantra, a retreat on this deity should start on the tenth or the twenty-fifth of the Tibetan month. These are special auspicious dates for tantric yoga, when there is much movement of the dakas and dakinis and your nervous system can easily be blessed. Because of the intensity of the daka-dakini energy at those times, you can discover everlasting blissful energy within the chakras of your nervous system simply through starting on either of these day,. For the same reason, it is best to start retreats on deities of the mother tantra class in the evening, after sunset.

SOME GENERAL PREPARATIONS

If you are doing retreat alone, you may need someone to help with the shopping and cooking. Your helper should be totally positive toward you and what you are doing, and you should have a good relationship with this person. If your helper thinks you are ridiculous or that what you are doing is evil, it will be a great disturbance to your mind. Similarly, if you are retreating with a group, it should not include people with whom you cannot get along. It is important that you create the best possible conditions for your retreat.

If you don't have a helper and are not in group retreat where eating arrangements are usually made for you, you should try to obtain most of the food you'll need for the duration of your retreat beforehand. Don't get too much; rather, limit yourself to basic things as much as possible. This is what we used to do in Tibet.

Before starting retreat you should cut your connections with the outside world and abandon whatever expectations you have of it. Although you are retreating in order to cut off your ignorance, this internal cutting is a gradual process that starts with your detaching yourself from the outside world. Therefore, you should abandon all expectations of visits from friends, letters, chocolates from your parents, and the like.

Furthermore, you must decide before your retreat starts who you will allow yourself to meet and how far from the place of retreat you can go. Thus, you might decide, "During this retreat I shall talk to my parents but to nobody else," or, "During this retreat I shall go as far as the spring to wash but no further." Such decisions are very helpful for your mind. In Tibetan we call it *tsam war gyu* ("putting retreat"), which means you'll meet certain people if necessary, but no others. The more outside people you meet the more samsaric information you collect, so instead of gaining wisdom you gain mental pollution.

Similarly, you must finish all your letter-writing and other business before you start, otherwise your retreat will constantly be disturbed by distracting thoughts of, "I have to do this," "I really should do that...." Make sure that while your body is in the retreat room, your mind doesn't wander back home.

Many Tibetan yogis would abandon the world for years—or even their whole lives—in order to ensure themselves of perfect retreat conditions.

Some even sealed themselves into doorless caves, receiving their food through a small hole in the wall.

One of the most important preparations is your determination to succeed. You should feel, "I am so fortunate to have received this perfect human life in which I have the opportunity of receiving the everlasting blissful realizations of Heruka Vajrasattva. Therefore, no matter what samsaric experiences I have during this retreat, be they good or bad, I shall control my mind." Thus, whether you experience samsaric happiness or difficulties, you do not over-react but take the middle way.

For example, one morning you might wake up with a headache and think that you are too sick to go to the session. A little headache won't kill you! You are here for retreat. That means you have to exercise control. You can meditate with a headache. Or perhaps a beautiful, ego-breaking present from your parents suddenly arrives, and you lose control and get very excited: "Wow! I've been waiting for this for more than a year; I must take it right away." You should not do this. Do not get excited. It doesn't matter; have control.

WHAT TO EAT

When you are doing a *kriya* tantra retreat, the food restrictions are quite strict. In a maha-anuttara yoga tantra retreat you have a bit more latitude but should still avoid what we call "black" foods—meat (especially chicken, pork, and fish), eggs, garlic, onions, and radish. Garlic is very heavy and disturbs your nervous system by either making it feel too full or causing too much movement within it. If the onions are not too strong, they're probably okay. The problem with radish is that it causes gas and makes you break wind.

Fruit and vegetables are good, and so are so-called "white" foods like milk, yogurt, and cheese, which are considered pure. You can also have muesli, chocolate, and even Vegemite, which despite its color is not a black food!

My advice is that you keep yourself as healthy as possible. Some people think, "Oh, I'm doing Dharma; I don't need anything." That's wrong. When you're in retreat trying to develop Dharma wisdom, it makes more sense to feed yourself even better than you normally do—and you know how much you usually give to take care of your samsaric body.

Sometimes retreaters experience so much bliss and joy in a session that they just want to keep going and not stop for food. This is your baby mind speaking—don't trust it. Take your meals as scheduled. But while breakfast and lunch are fine, there's a question about whether or not you should eat dinner. It's better to avoid eating in the evening because a full stomach impairs concentration. It depends on the individual. We're all different: some people can eat only a little at a time; for them, I'd say dinner is okay. Those who can manage a good breakfast and lunch should keep the evening meal very light or, preferably, skip it altogether. Be flexible; food is not all that important. Just stay healthy.

Sometimes people take the eight Mahayana precepts during retreat.[8] On those days, of course, you can't have breakfast or dinner. You can choose whether to take them every day or not; it's up to you. In my opinion, the best days to take them are the full and new moon days. Taking precepts gives you great energy and is another excellent way of taking action to purify yourself.

CLEANING THE RETREAT PLACE

Since you are going to clean yourself inside, you should also make the outside clean. Your retreat room should be exceptionally clean and very neat and tidy. Do not leave things hanging or lying all over the place; their disorderly vibration will only agitate your mind. Nor should you distract your mind by having objects of attachment in your room. No animals, including dogs, should be allowed to enter. After cleaning your room, you can sprinkle saffron, sandalwood, rose water, or any other kind of perfume around so that it smells beautiful and not a trace of any bad odor remains. Instead of putting perfume on your body with attachment, put it around the retreat room so that just walking into the room is a completely blissful experience. You should also sprinkle some blessed inner offering nectar around the room. Do all this before you start retreat and every morning as well.

THE MEDITATION SEAT

The next thing to do is to arrange your meditation seat. It should be as comfortable as possible, so much so that you feel that you could sit there for twenty-four hours without a break, experiencing only bliss. The seat should not be flat; you should have a small pillow beneath your buttocks so that they are higher than your knees. This will help you keep your back straight and prevent you from getting pins and needles in your legs. A thin, lumpy, uncomfortable seat does not necessarily signify renunciation.

Beneath the seat there should be a right-pointing swastika drawn on the floor in chalk or rice, or on a piece of paper. The swastika is an ancient Indian symbol of auspiciousness. The word comes from the Sanskrit *svasti,* which means well-being. It also symbolizes the indestructible, or vajra, seat that Buddha sat upon at Bodhgaya when he became enlightened. It is not easy to reach enlightenment; you can't get enlightened just anywhere. The buddhas of this fortunate eon attain enlightenment at Bodhgaya. Since we ourselves are retreating in order to reach enlightenment, we too should have a vajra seat, not an up-and-down, here-today-gone-tomorrow, yo-yo seat. If you're in a boat, you automatically go up and down with the ocean. Your meditation seat should not be like that. Since we cannot put an actual vajra beneath our seat, we use this symbolic representation. The combination of an indestructible seat with an indestructible, pure, enlightened attitude makes your retreat really worthwhile.

You can also put two kinds of grass under your seat. One is *kusha* grass, the grass that some Indian brooms are made of. There are two bits of this arranged so that their tips point in toward the center of the swastika from the back, their stems pointing backward. At Bodhgaya, Buddha sat on a cushion of kusha grass. Using the same grass reminds us of Lord Buddha's meditation experiences, especially his making the decision to remain seated on that grass until he reached enlightenment, no matter how difficult it was or how many hardships he had to bear. Kusha grass is composed of hundreds of slender strands, all lying parallel, orderly, close together, and pointing the one way. It symbolizes strong, single-pointed concentration and clear visualization—all your energy flowing in the one direction.

The other kind of grass is called *tsa dur-wa* in Tibetan; it is like couch or *kikuyu* grass. This is arranged in the same way as the kusha grass, two bits pointing in toward the center of the swastika from the back. The pieces you use should have as many joints as possible. This type of grass is considered auspicious for a long life.

Once you have arranged your seat you cannot move it for any reason whatsoever. Westerners always want to shake out their cushions or leave them in the sun, but in retreat this is not allowed. You also cannot move your seat to another part of the room once the retreat has started. You have to control your schizophrenic mind.

In a group retreat there should be plenty of space between one person and the next. You don't have to squash up like Tibetans in puja. I remember a student once having trouble because he had put his seat down on a damp section of the floor and his small carpet became moldy and rotted. Therefore, you should be careful at the beginning, when you are first deciding where to put your seat.

At home, also, you should try to have a special meditation seat, preferably not in your bedroom, which tends to have a strong samsaric vibration. If you can set up a shrine in a separate room or in a quiet corner of your house and use that only for meditation, it will help you a lot. The Dharma trip and the samsara trip are completely different—unless you have a great realization of bodhicitta, they don't go together at all.

In front of you there should be a small table for your vajra (*dorje*), bell (*drilbu*), *damaru,* kapala and, if you need it, sadhana text. The kapala contains the inner offering liquid, which is usually black tea with a special, blessed inner offering pill dissolved in it. However, in a group retreat it is not necessary that everyone have these things. It's enough if just one or two of the retreaters have them. If you don't have an actual dorje and bell, a drawing of them will do.

The Rosary

You should have a special rosary that you use only in retreats and do not allow other people to see. Some retreats require you to use a rosary made of bone or some other specific substance. It should not be worn around your wrist or neck but treated with respect. Once the retreat has started, you cannot take the rosary out of the room and should leave it on your table. You must never take your rosary into the bathroom. Before the retreat starts, the rosary should be blessed by a lama, and each morning, at the beginning of the first session, you should bless it yourself with the mantra OM RUTSIRA MANI PRAWA TAYA HUM. Say this mantra seven times and blow on the rosary.

Arranging the Altar

After you have cleaned the room, arrange your altar. Put your image of Heruka Vajrasattva on the altar, or if it is a picture hang it on the wall above. You should not put other images on your altar. During this retreat Heruka Vajrasattva is the most important deity—your manifestation of universal reality—and you don't need any others.

Ideally, you should use three different offering cakes (*tormas*).[9] In Tibet we used to make these out of roasted barley flour (*tsampa*), but in the West you can use chocolate, candy, biscuits, cake, or other foods instead.

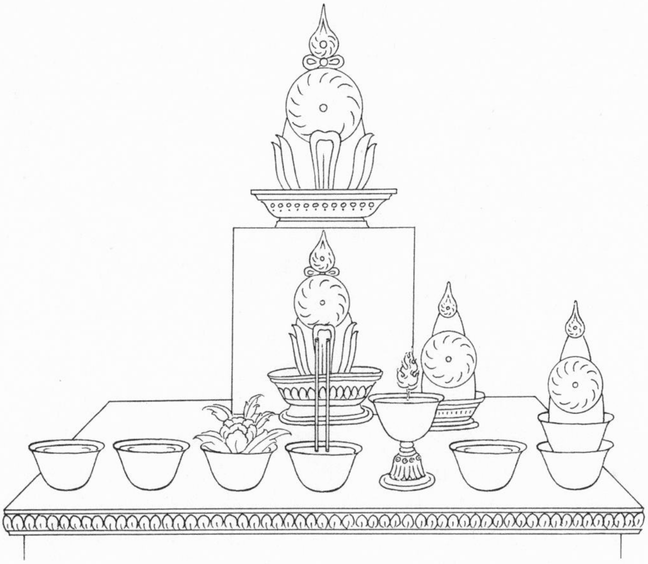

Drawing by Peter Iseli

The main torma (shown at the top) is your offering to Heruka Vajrasattva. You bless it with the blissful transcendental wisdom of Vajrasattva through the methods of tantric yoga and leave it on your altar until the end of your retreat.[10] When we make this out of tsampa we usually add a little alcohol, which by nature has the energy of expansion and development, to symbolize the meditator's development of kundalini energy through the yoga method.[11] The second torma (shown immediately below the first) is for the special wrathful protector of Heruka, whose job is to pacify all uncontrolled energy. Once you have put it on your altar you should not remove it until you have finished your retreat.[12]

Thirdly, no matter where you retreat, there will be local deities, or spirits (*shi-dak*), who possess or control that place. In order to prevent them from taking offense at your intrusion onto their property and giving you harm, it is necessary to make an offering to them. Again, this does not have to be a Tibetan torma (as shown just to the right of the second torma above) but can be rice or any of the other things mentioned before. It also stays on your altar for the duration of your retreat.[13] Visualize your offering as whatever those sentient beings need and would enjoy, and feel that you are also offering your body and speech to these beings, sacrificing yourself for the sake of *all* sentient beings.

As you make the offering think, "Please let me do here what I have to do: purify myself and gain wisdom and compassion for the sake of all sentient beings. I am not trying to take this place away from you, but just using it for a short time. Therefore, please do not worry or be angry, jealous, or afraid. Please have compassion, help me, and do not interfere. Take this offering and whatever else you need." Visualize that the spirits take the offering, are very happy and satisfied, and give you permission to use the place in safety. In the Hinayana sutras Buddha explained that before a monastery is built permission should be sought from the spirits who own the land, trees, and other things at that place. If we do not make these offerings, the spirits may get angry and harm us physically or mentally. Even if they are unable to harm us by day, they can cause us to have bad dreams or disturb us in other ways at night.

Offering bowls, candles, butter lamps or other light offerings, flowers, and food should also be offered on your altar. Change the water and make fresh light and incense offerings before each session. The light you offer symbolizes the inner light of wisdom that you are trying to develop; incense represents your pure morality.

Why do we offer so much water? It's not because Vajrasttava is always thirsty; there's no such thing as a deity actually taking your offerings. No, the problem is our miserliness. We usually give with the spirit of attachment; this sneaky spirit is somehow completely unified with our gift. So when you offer water, it's so freely available that you don't grasp at it, and in this way you get used to giving without attachment or expectation. Therefore, offering water is very useful: it costs you nothing, and you get great benefit for just a little work. Also, water has many precious qualities; and it contains the energy of all kinds of precious jewels within.[14] Bless the water you offer with the mantra OM AH HUM, which symbolizes Vajrasattva's enlightened body, speech, and mind. Thus, although it looks like you're putting water on your altar, in fact, because of the blessed transformation, you are offering the blissful nectar of transcendental wisdom and compassion.

As I mentioned before, it is highly beneficial to make physical offerings as often as you can. The lazy mind will say, "Real offerings are internal; I don't need to go through the ritual of making all these external offerings on the altar." Don't give in to laziness—it is much better for you to engage in the action of giving. Unless, I'm going to say, you are completely in samadhi. That's the only exception I'm going to make. Spending your time absorbed in single-pointed concentration may be more important. But when you have plenty of time to do other things but no time to make a decent altar, it shows how misconceived your samsaric value judgments really are.

Also, a small portion of your food or drink should be blessed and offered on the altar before you take it yourself. Offer a little of your morning tea in a small bowl, a portion of your lunch on a plate. This is very useful for loosening attachment and developing the perfection of generosity.

At the end of the day, the food you have offered can be taken off the altar and eaten the next day. Also, you do not have to restrict your offerings to the material ones I have been talking about. You can transform them mentally into infinite offerings of the best kinds of nectar, flowers, incense, lights, perfumes, food, sound, and so forth, and along with these offer everything else in the universe transformed into sublime blissful offerings, as we do when we offer a mandala.

All these practices may not be the most important thing you can do, but they are very useful in your spiritual development.

8

The Retreat Session

The daily schedule

In general, it is best to start your retreat with short sessions of an hour's duration at the most. These are recommended because if a session is short, you will do it well. Sessions in which you are alert and your concentration is strong are obviously better than ones in which your mind is tired and sleepy. We have been asleep for countless lives, now it's time to wake up!

It is said that the length of sessions throughout a retreat should resemble the shape of a grain of barley: pointed at the ends and wide in the middle. Thus, sessions at the beginning and end of a retreat should be short and those in the middle longer. As your retreat progresses and your meditation gains in strength, you gradually increase the length of the sessions. Toward the end of the retreat, as you prepare to face the world once more, you shorten them again. If you do not do this and finish your retreat still doing long intensive sessions, there is the danger of your first contact with the outside world upsetting you or making you sick. The vibration will be too different from what you have been experiencing.

Short sessions give you much energy. You do not want to stop meditating when the session reaches an end. But you should. If you stop meditating only when you are exhausted, you will have no enthusiasm for the next session. The mere sight of your meditation cushion will nauseate you. This is obviously not good. Or, as I mentioned before, sometimes you might feel so blissful and energetic that you just want to keep on meditating all day. But if you do that, it is almost certain that the next day you will feel the exact opposite and not want to meditate at all. Gradually increasing the length of your sessions ensures that you always finish with an alert mind eager for more meditation. Treat your baby mind wisely.

One Tibetan lama recommended eighteen sessions a day! Perhaps we could settle for about eight to start with. Get up early enough to ensure that your first session finishes before sunrise. Take a coffee break and do another session before breakfast. Between breakfast and lunch you can do two more sessions separated by a fifteen minute break. After lunch you can rest, work, study teachings on the graduated path or the Heruka Vajrasattva commentary, or do your daily commitments or other meditations. Then you can do two more sessions separated by a fifteen minute break before afternoon tea. After that you do another session, have dinner, and do the final session of the day. The best time to conduct a discussion group is after lunch, before the first afternoon session. It should definitely not be after or instead of the last session of the day. That is the wrong time to stimulate discursive thought. Of course, all this is just a rough guide. Naturally, as sessions get longer, there will be fewer each day.

By the middle of the retreat you could be doing four sessions a day: one before sunrise, one between breakfast and lunch, one between lunch and dinner and the last one after that. However, you should not be in session at sunrise, noon, sunset or midnight. At those times the changes in the vibrations of the external environment affect your nervous system, automatically causing your mind to be distracted. Therefore, you should avoid meditating during these periods.

Tibetan monks would rise at two or three in the morning when in retreat; but in hot countries it is difficult to do without sleep and also, you are not used to this kind of discipline. If you get up too early, you will get tired very easily and that will spoil your meditation. You should keep healthy and do your sleeping in bed, not on your meditation cushion. Whatever you do, do well.

In conclusion, then, it is best not to push yourself unreasonably. You cannot imitate Milarepa—don't even try. Be comfortable and relaxed, take your retreat easy, and make it worthwhile.

JUST BEFORE THE SESSION

Washing. Before each session you should clean your teeth and wash your body. If you cannot wash your whole body, you should at least wash your face, neck, arms, armpits, and feet. This will prevent your mind from getting sluggish and sleepy during the session. Having washed, you wake up, feel more comfortable, and are able to meditate with fully awakened wisdom.

Coming on time. Make sure that you come into the meditation room at least five minutes before the start of the session, especially if it is your job to arrange the altar. Do not come rushing in, out of breath, puffing and sweating just as the session is about to begin. Come in slowly and mindfully, do three prostrations, and sit down gently. Collect and calm your mind. Think: "On this seat I shall purify myself completely in order to attain the enlightened state of Vajrasattva for the sake of all mother sentient beings." Then, with awareness, purify your nervous system with the blessed inner offering. Dip the tip of the ring finger of your left hand into the inner offering in your kapala, touch it to your tongue, and feel the blessed energy flowing throughout your nervous system, purifying it of all negativity and filling you with blissful wisdom.

Do not disturb others. Do not talk to the members of your group when you come into the meditation room or disturb them in any other way. It is good if you can keep the meditation room an area of total silence for the duration of the retreat. If you have things to do in the room, such as cleaning or arranging the altar, do them without involving others.

Arranging the altar. As I said before, make fresh offerings before each session. I recommend that in a group retreat you make an offering of five candles or butter lamps each time. Make your offerings with the pure, sincere thought that, "I am making this offering for the everlasting blissful divine wisdom of Heruka Vajrasattva to grow within me so that I will be able to lead all mother sentient beings to the discovery of this realization in their own minds."

BEGINNING THE SESSION

I mentioned silence in the meditation room before, but once the session begins, there must be absolutely no talking. Start by taking refuge and generating bodhicitta with the prayers in the sadhana, but remember what I said before: taking refuge and generating bodhicitta are states of mind beyond words; make sure your mind becomes one with them. When the prayers finish, do not go straight on to the breath-holding exercise, but stay a while in meditation on refuge and bodhicitta. If you combine these attitudes with your mind properly at the beginning of the session, their energy will carry through until the end and pervade your entire practice, making it far more beneficial.

SESSIONS IN GENERAL

I have already stressed the great importance of single-pointed concentration during recitation of the mantra. This cannot be over-emphasized. Most of the time our minds are fully occupied by superstitions and wrong conceptions, and everything we do is under their influence. It is most important that at least while we are in retreat, we do not allow them to arise for even a moment, otherwise we shall not receive the realizations that we seek. Therefore, be very careful to ensure that for the duration of the retreat your mind is completely free of these delusions. This is even more important with respect to the session, and crucial while you are reciting the mantra.

You must also avoid other disturbances to the session, such as talking, eating, getting up from your seat, and leaving the room to go to the toilet, or for any other reason. Make sure you go to the toilet before the start of the session.

The great ancient yogi Phadampa Sanggye said that there are five things to which you have to pay special attention if you want to do a perfect retreat. He said that if you do not take care of these, your retreat will become almost useless.

The first is the *power of body*. During the session you must maintain your visualization of the deity continuously. If you lose it and allow your wrong conceptions' samsaric projection of yourself to arise—"I am so-and-so; I am hungry and thirsty"—you have lost the power of body. The second is the *power of speech*. If you speak during the session, you have directly interrupted this power. Next is the *power of mind*. You lose it as soon as your single-pointed concentration is broken. The fourth is the *power of signs*. During retreat there are signs that appear in your mind. If you come into contact with people who are not in retreat, this power is lost. Finally, there is the *power of energy*: there are negative repercussions from letting people who are not in your retreat see the image of your deity or the blessed way in which you eat. Therefore, you must not allow them to do so.

We also talk about body, speech, and mind retreats. *Body retreat* means that you cut the connection with your deluded projections of your body. Also, during retreat you are not allowed to lose the power of your body. For example, when you are meditating on a samadhi female, you must not lose semen.

Speech retreat means that you avoid any ordinary conversation, which only induces agitation in your mind. You must retain the power of speech, which will be explained when we discuss mantra recitation. You are not even allowed to spit.

Mind retreat means that you cut off all superstitions, the actions of the deluded mind. You keep the power of your mind by preventing any deluded, superstitious thoughts from entering.

THE SADHANA

This book contains the Heruka Vajrasattva sadhana [see appendix 1] that I have compiled for the purpose of retreat. You can do it in English or Tibetan. If you do it in Tibetan, make sure you have the translation handy so that you will understand the meaning. You can do it in English, but somehow the Tibetan has a very good feeling and some kind of blessed energy associated with it.[15]

MANTRA RECITATION

The mantra of Heruka Vajrasattva is extremely powerful. Reciting it even once shakes your negativities to their very foundation. However, for it to be effective, you must say it very clearly; one mantra recited with perfect sound has more power than a hundred mumbled ones. By perfect sound I mean that each syllable should be articulated distinctly: cleanly, clearly, and smoothly, with a uniform rhythm and pitch. It should not be slurred or irregular, with some phrases fast and others slow, or some syllables high and others low. Therefore, pay close attention to this point. When you recite the mantra, you more or less whisper it quietly, so that you can hear it yourself, but the person sitting next to you cannot. Make sure your recitation doesn't disturb others.

If you do this mantra properly—with single-pointed concentration and clear visualization—it really becomes transcendental and transforms your body into the bliss-pervaded divine body, your speech into divine blissful speech, and your mind into divine blissful wisdom. If, on the other hand, your mind is occupied by negative energy, there is not much power in your retreat and everything remains ordinary. Therefore, you should know which factors that, in addition to unclear recitation, prevent your mantra from becoming transcendental.

You should not say the mantra too loudly, too softly, too quickly, or too slowly. To keep you aware and to ensure that the mantras you count in your tally have all been said correctly, there are a number of penalties that you incur when certain faults interrupt your session. Thus, if you leave the room or even get up out of your seat or speak, you cannot count any of the mantras of that session. Ideally, once the session starts you should not move your legs at all. If you fall asleep, drop your rosary, lose concentration, get angry, or find yourself saying the wrong mantra, you cannot count any of the mantras that you have recited on that round of the rosary. You have to go back to the first bead and start all over again. Losing concentration is one of the worst faults. All of a sudden you find that your mind has wandered back to your home, into a supermarket, to a meeting with your friend...you must not allow this kind of thing to happen.

If you break wind, there is a penalty of seven mantras: you have to go back seven rosary beads and continue from there. Similarly, there is a penalty of five if you cough, sneeze, clear your throat, blow your nose, hiccup, or belch during recitation of the mantra. The mantra blesses your speech and breath, and you should not waste this precious energy. That means you should also avoid wasting your breath by blowing out candles and lamps, blowing on fires, whistling, and so forth during your retreat.

There are two ways of deciding the length of a retreat: by time or by number of mantras. The length of a Vajrasattva retreat is usually three months or the time it takes to recite one hundred thousand mantras. Actually, you should add ten percent of the number of mantras you are committed to do in any retreat to compensate for those recited badly. Thus in a Vajrasattva retreat you should recite one hundred and ten thousand mantras.[16] This can usually be done in three months.

The problem with having a commitment to do a certain number of mantras is that you get obsessed by the "score," and this disturbs the peace of your retreat. It is better to do fewer mantras properly than more in a sloppy fashion. And, of course, you can count toward the total only full rosaries of mantra and the mantras you recite in session, not those done during the breaks.

I remember once being in a group retreat of one hundred monks in our refugee camp in West Bengal. We were committed to counting a certain number of mantras, and the retreat could not finish until each monk had completed his total. One of the monks had great trouble articulating the mantra and by the time the rest of us had finished he still had a long way to go. He was so embarrassed that he could not show his face, and sat with his head covered by his robes while he recited the remaining mantras. We had to sit there for about five days waiting for him to finish! I don't think he should have reacted like that. Just counting a certain number of mantras is not the point. You can do some other meditation instead. The important thing is to take advantage of the retreat situation and do what suits your individual needs.[17]

ENDING THE SESSION

At the end of the sadhana, just before the dedication, Heruka Vajrasattva dissolves into you and you become one with him. At this time, it would be good to do a short glance meditation on the graduated path, such as Lama Tsong Khapa's *Three Principles of the Path, Concise Meaning of the Stages of the Path,* or *The Foundation of All Excellence,* all of which can be found in Geshe Wangyel's book, *The Door of Liberation.* In a group retreat, the leader reads out the meditation and everybody else meditates. After that, you dedicate your merits. Your dedication at the end of the last session of the day should be particularly strong. Then, remain seated for a few more minutes, single-pointedly contemplating your blissful unity with Heruka Vajrasattva's holy body, speech, and mind, not allowing a single dualistic thought to arise.

9

More Retreat Advice

Between sessions

For the serious retreater the session breaks are just as important as the sessions themselves. Actually, session breaks should *be* sessions. You put so much effort into creating a beautiful environment in the meditation room and developing your mind during the sessions; make sure that between sessions you do not destroy all that you have gained. During the sessions you have good concentration and feel blissful, but when you come out, you become unaware and ordinary. You are like someone who walks along a sandy beach trying to smooth out his footprints as he goes, while making new ones all the time. You should not feel, therefore, that your sessions are heaven and the breaks are hell.

During the session, while you are concentrating well on the deity, your mundane thoughts cannot intrude, and for that time your mind is free of them. You should maintain such concentrated awareness after the session, too. In this way you can totally eliminate your samsaric mind. The old habits are there, waiting for the chance to arise, so you have to be mindful not to give in to them.

The short breaks should last at least fifteen minutes so that you have a chance to get some exercise; walk, stretch your legs, and relax your body. However, do not relax your gentle awareness; try to keep your mind even and stable, at the level you attained during the session. This is relatively easy in the short breaks, but much more difficult in the longer ones—at mealtimes and at night. Therefore, you should take the opportunity of the short breaks to practice this kind of session break meditation.

As I said before, at the end of the session, Heruka Vajrasattva dissolves into you, you become inseparably one with him, and before you get up and leave the room, you sit for a few minutes or more meditating on this blissful union, your body, speech, and mind being one with Heruka

Vajrasattva's holy body, speech, and mind. You should have the clear appearance of yourself as the deity and the divine pride of *being* Vajrasattva himself. This is the concentration that you must maintain between sessions. You must never think, "I am so-and-so; I am a such-and-such from here or there," as your ego habitually projects. As soon as you start to think like this, problems begin. If you cannot maintain the thought, "I am Heruka Vajrasattva," you should at least think, "I must attain the divine state of Heruka Vajrasattva as quickly as possible for the sole purpose of enlightening all sentient beings."

Throughout the retreat you should feel highly fortunate to have the chance of practicing this highest tantric yoga method and actualizing the six transcendental perfections for the sake of all sentient beings. Realize with joy that for almost the first time in your life you are doing something truly meaningful. If you analyze your life honestly you will see that most of it has been spent in efforts to satisfy your hallucinating, craving mind with illusory objects of the senses. Your dualistic wrong conceptions have never given you the time or space to exercise your wisdom.

From the moment you wake, craving for coffee and other objects of the senses, to the moment you sleep, craving the pleasure of unconsciousness, your day is filled with actions motivated by ignorant, grasping attachment. You enjoy without awareness the few small pleasures that you find and believe that the illusory projections of your dualistic mind and the perceptions of your defiled senses are reality itself. Not for a moment do you allow your wisdom to function. Thus goes your life and thus it finishes, in misery.

Now that you have the chance to do something about all this, it is imperative that you do not waste a moment. Therefore, you must remain aware throughout the entire day, not only during sessions. If you feel that the time in the sessions is Dharma and that when you are eating, you are in samsara, there is something wrong with your understanding. What makes tantric yoga so powerful is that it gives no time for samsara. There is no way that a proper tantric practitioner can say at one moment, "Now I'm practicing Dharma," and at another, "Now my actions are samsaric." Tantra contains all the methods required to transform every single action into Dharma wisdom.

If you believe that meditation is Dharma and eating, drinking, shopping, and so forth are samsara, you will never be able to attain liberation.

The amount of time you spend for what you believe to be Dharma, the path to liberation—meditation—will be negligible in comparison to the rest. However, if you are skillful in your application of wisdom and method, everything you do, even the things you consider to be worldly, can become the path to enlightenment. Thus, your whole life becomes tantric yoga, and there is no space for samsara. Once you have stopped your samsaric mind from functioning, how is it possible that you will not quickly attain perfect liberation?

In the Paramitayana, desire is considered bad. The Vinaya says, "You cannot do this; you must not touch that." Sometimes you feel that you cannot have even a drop of water. The powerful methods of tantric yoga take desire as just another resource on the rapid path to enlightenment. You transform any pleasures that you have into experiences of the blissful wisdom of the deity. You should not feel guilty because you are enjoying the things you have or because others don't have them. That does not help anybody.

Enjoy with bliss whatever you do. When you eat and drink, bless the food and drink with the mantra OM AH HUM, thereby transforming it into the nature of the holy body, speech, and mind of Heruka Vajrasattva, and offer it to yourself identified as the deity. Feel the blissful energy of the blessed substances pervade your entire nervous system. If you do this with wisdom, it can help to quickly bring you the realizations of transcendental bliss. If you eat and drink only with desire and interpret the experience in an ordinary way, you have a very samsaric experience. It all depends upon your mind. When you go to sleep, do not allow your ego's projection of yourself to arise, but sleep feeling blissfully one with Heruka Vajrasattva. When you wash, visualize yourself as Vajrasattva and think, "Heruka Vajrasattva's holy body is free from all defilements, but I am washing to purify my dualistic mind."

Your usual view of yourself is projected by your ego. Between sessions you have to recognize yourself instead as the manifestation of blissful transcendental wisdom, Heruka Vajrasattva. Thus, whatever you perceive is the view of this non-dual mind and in the nature of non-duality. In this sphere of non-duality the whole world passes by. You feel that it is almost like a television show. The world no longer has its usual concrete appearance and, therefore, cannot disturb you. It seems like an illusion or a dream. Thus, you should determine that whatever appears to your senses is not real, contrary to what you have always believed. Whenever you see others, you should see them not in their ordinary form but in the aspect of Heruka Vajrasattva and treat them with the utmost respect.

RETREAT IN GENERAL

You may have thought that retreat was easy. I am sure that by now you can see that if done properly, it is not. However, it is worth doing strictly; the stricter your retreat, the better the results you can obtain. Retreat is the only way to really transform your mind, because in retreat you are putting the teachings into action, not merely collecting more information. With transformation, the solution to your problems comes. You yourself become the Heruka Vajrasattva method meditation instead of you being *here*, looking at the printed sadhana *there*. When there is that kind of separation, there is the danger that your mind will start telling you, "You are a Westerner; this is Tibetan…why are you doing this?" All sorts of doubts will arise. When you practice and achieve results, there is no doubt.

Therefore, you should do your retreat as strictly as possible, keeping your mind in the sphere of the transcendental process continuously. Sitting in a cave while your mind keeps wandering back home is not being in retreat. Your body, speech, and mind should be focused on the same thing. Most of the time your mind is split and agitated, and you cannot do mundane things without coming down from a state of higher awareness. In retreat you must learn how to unify the two—the mundane and the transcendent.

Our minds are somewhat crazy and out of control, therefore, we need to treat them firmly. But the strict discipline of a retreat is entirely different from the external control that is often forced on mentally disturbed people in the West. You cannot bring about a fundamental change in a person's mind through institutionalization, electric shocks, drug therapy, or indoctrination. It must instead be done voluntarily, gently, and skillfully. Sometimes retreaters themselves are unskillful. They imagine that they are great ascetic meditators and want to become famous as such. They change their appearance and push themselves until their nervous systems explode. You cannot change your mind as simply as you can change the color of your clothes by dyeing them. Discipline yourselves wisely.

Thus, if you want your retreat to be successful, you should have the right attitude toward it. You should not feel that it is some kind of prison sentence, during which you are going to be locked up for a certain period, unable to go to the movies, see your friends, converse freely, and so forth. Instead you should feel joyful and fortunate that at last you have the chance to do something highly beneficial for yourself and others, a rare opportunity that you have not had before and may not have again. All the same, you should not have the expectation, "This is incredible. Heruka Vajrasattva is going to appear to me and say, 'My son…my daughter….'" This is unrealistic and becomes a hindrance to your meditation. You should be relaxed yet have the strong determination that, "On this seat I am going to actualize the yoga method of Heruka Vajrasattva. Until I have received the signs of success I shall not break this retreat."

To give yourself the best chance of success you must reduce distractions to the minimum. You have to create an environment that suits your needs. When you do worldly business, you set up your office in a certain way. Now your business is retreat, and you should act accordingly. The meditation room should be comfortable, clean, and very tidy. Similarly, the room in which you sleep should not be decorated with pictures or other objects that stimulate your delusions. You should avoid meeting or talking to outside people as much as possible. The news they bring and their vibration can only disturb your concentration. It is best not to talk to even the other people in your retreat until lunchtime, and then the conversation should be only about Dharma, not all your past experiences, future plans, or other gossip. If you are feeling very tense and need to talk to relax, as a kind of therapy, perhaps that is acceptable, but you should be careful not to waste your own energy or that of others.

You should not write or receive letters. Even if your best friend suddenly turns up unexpectedly, you should not meet him or her; remember, before the retreat starts you have to decide strictly whom you will and will not meet, keeping outsiders to a minimum. If there is something urgent or important to say, you can write a note. If a beautiful present arrives, you should not accept it until the retreat has finished. You should be careful what you read in retreat and avoid all samsaric literature completely: newspapers, magazines, novels, technical books, poetry, and astrological charts.

Even certain Dharma books should be avoided during retreat. Those that deal with philosophical doctrine are too dry and intellectual and may only add to your confusion and superstitions instead of enhancing the psychological treatment that retreat is supposed to be. But you can read books on the graduated path or commentaries on the yoga method; however, even these should not be read too much. Read only books that help you. Doing glance meditation on the graduated path during the breaks is especially useful because it directs your energy into the right channel. Sometimes in retreat your mind can veer toward extremes; the graduated path can bring you back to center.

There are many other disciplines that have been found helpful for preserving the pure energy of retreat. You should not take things in and out of the meditation room, especially your rosary and ritual implements, such as your vajra and bell, and people not in retreat and animals should not enter it. You should not allow others to sleep in your bed or sit on your meditation seat. You cannot take your seat outside to air or clean it; all you can do is brush it off. You should not touch weapons, such as guns or bombs, or put knives, arrows, and so forth in your mouth. You should not use others' plates, cups, or cutlery or allow them to use yours. And one of the worst things you can do is to fight with other members of the group. That really breaks the retreat.

There are also many things that you can do during retreat. In a group, "karma yoga" is good. Each person has a little work to do, helping the Dharma center or serving the other members. However, all this should be worked out before the retreat starts and rosters drawn up so that everyone knows what his or her job is and there is not too much discussion about it once the retreat has started. Thus, people are needed to clean the meditation room and arrange the altar before each session. Help may be needed in the kitchen or with serving food. Some people might like to do some gardening. Others might like to transcribe tapes or edit teachings for publication. These activities are good and help keep you balanced, but while doing them, you must maintain the mindfulness that I have already described.

During the breaks you can also do other practices: your daily commitments, prostrations, and so forth. You can also recite Vajrasattva mantras, but remember, these don't count toward your retreat total.

One of the most important things you can do to ensure the success of your retreat is to stay healthy. Some people equate retreat with what they imagine to be asceticism: uncomfortable conditions, an unhealthy environment, poor food, feeling hungry and thirsty, not sleeping, wearing rags, and so forth. This is completely wrong. First, these are not the signs of asceticism. Second, as I said before, tantric yoga has the methods of transforming all pleasures and comforts into the rapid path to enlightenment. Therefore, as long as you can use it wisely, you can have whatever you like. You should stay in a clean, healthy place, have a beautiful blissful room, a comfortable seat, a good place to sleep, and plenty of good food.

Treat yourself with respect—after all, you are Heruka Vajrasattva! Offer yourself nice clothes and eat well. That does not mean you should overeat. If you eat too much you will not be able to meditate. The food you eat should be clean and healthy. You should not accept food from people suffering from contagious diseases, like tuberculosis. And as I mentioned before, it is better to avoid "black" foods such as meat, eggs, onions, garlic, and radish, and it is essential to do so if your retreat is from the kriya class of tantra. Otherwise there is not much restriction on the type of food you can eat. Some people like to fast during retreat. In a long retreat you should fast with moderation.

If you do not eat properly, there is the danger that your nervous system and the energy winds of your body will become disturbed. A strong retreat itself has the tendency to do this, and a poor diet compounds the risk. Such disturbances manifest as nervous breakdowns, "spacing out," or physical pains, especially in the heart chakra. Sometimes you will get pain in the heart because your visualization of the nectar that rushes down from Vajrasattva's heart into your central channel is too concrete. You are concentrating strongly at your heart and think that something physical is hitting it. This is a fundamental error, but it is much easier to develop such symptoms if you do not take care of your health.

Be kind to yourself. When you do a good session, pat yourself on the back and congratulate yourself. Offer yourself good food as a reward! If you do badly, scold yourself gently and make yourself promise to try harder. Make sure you get enough sleep. It is much better to sleep properly at night and do strong sessions than to fall asleep while trying to meditate.

If you experience many hindrances during your retreat, you can do a Mahakala protector puja or emphasize meditation on sunyata, which is actually the best protection. You should recognize bad signs and bad dreams as illusory and not take them seriously. Anyway, keep a written record of whatever good or bad experiences you have. Later, this will be useful both for yourself, as a reminder of what happened in your retreat, and for others who will be doing this retreat in future.

If you do this retreat conscientiously, observing all the strict conditions laid out above, it is guaranteed that you will receive signs of realization. The various parts of the sadhana have been specifically arranged to lead your mind gradually, so that when you reach the mantra recitation, it is naturally concentrated. You cannot jump straight into single-pointedness; you have to build up to it. If you do this properly and observe all the other disciplines described, there will be signs—if not during the day, then in your dreams at night. Not that you should be expecting them. As I said before, just relax in the certainty that for once you are extracting the essence from your precious human life, and feel highly fortunate to be doing something that is not dedicated to samsaric pleasure. Then, do your best without pushing yourself. When signs come, be detached, steady, and controlled, and do not grasp at them emotionally. Do not tell others about or make a big show of your realizations. Be simple, humble, down-to-earth, and practical. Life is much easier that way.

Group retreat

My observations of Western students over many years have shown that when they do group retreats, they are more successful than when they retreat alone. This may not apply to all students, but it certainly does to most. Especially when students are new to retreat, or when the retreat is a long one of, say, three months, it is better to retreat with a group. When you are alone, it is too easy not to follow the schedule. One day your meditation might be going well, so you will try to meditate all day and not stick to the sessions. The next day you will be down and unable to do any meditation. Or one morning you will feel tired and skip the first session to sleep in. Or your leg or head might hurt, so again you'll make some excuse not to go. These things do not happen when you are a member of a group. You have a responsibility to the others to attend all sessions.

In a group retreat everybody benefits from shared energy: you help each other. If you are feeling depressed you consult your friend, whose sympathetic advice brings you up again. When someone else is having some difficulty that you have experienced and overcome, you can explain what should be done. We are not completely stupid and can be of significant help to each other. Therefore, I recommend group retreat until you have had enough experience to retreat alone.

CONCLUSION

If you get the chance—or make the time—to retreat, you are extremely fortunate. Few things are as beneficial as that. With strong renunciation of samsara, you have realized that you have been everywhere, done everything, and that it's useless doing the same old things again and again, getting absolutely nowhere. That stops your mind from wandering. If you find yourself in retreat dreaming of your hometown or some other desirable place, you can tell yourself, "I know what I'll do if I go back there. I've been doing it for lifetimes. Essentially, there's nothing new. Why keep getting caught in that old, uncontrolled samsaric trip?"

Therefore, by recognizing the nature of samsara and having the enthusiastic determination to completely cut its root, you have no expectation of pleasure from worldly things. Even if your best friend shows up, "Hey, come on! Let's go out and have a great time," you can say, "Wait a minute. Sorry. I've had enough of all that."

You're not just emotionally pushing yourself into some small hut and locking yourself in. Rather, with strong wisdom, you are really renouncing samsara. You know the sort of nonsense you're likely to get involved in with your family and friends, so you generate the strong motivation: "I'm not going to break this retreat until I have unified my body, speech, and mind with those of Heruka Vajrasattva."

We often do things halfheartedly. This is because our minds are split. When opposing mental tendencies come into conflict, we are susceptible to a nervous breakdown. So you really need to know very clearly why you are retreating and to make sure that your motivation is strong. You should feel that it is necessary and worthwhile, and that you are extremely fortunate to have the opportunity to do it: "I am so blessed to have the chance of to spend a couple of months in retreat, acting for once under the strong influence of wisdom instead of constantly running from one thing to another, touching honey." Do you know what I mean by touching honey? When you touch honey, it tends to stick to your fingers and to everything else you touch, making a mess, and it is very difficult to get rid of. Samsaric actions are a lot like that.

Therefore, start your retreat with great determination and no expectations: "It doesn't matter whether or not I receive all the realizations of enlightenment. It's enough that I am trying to control my mind and relax myself in this peaceful, tranquil atmosphere." To reach this conclusion just once is a result of great fortune. All samsaric trips are such a complete waste of time; they produce only more and more problems. If you are deeply aware of the nature of samsaric life, you will have no obstacles or distractions during your retreat. But if you are half-half, your mind will wander and bother you constantly: "Oh, if I were back home, I could be going out to dinner and the movies with my girlfriend…."

To the samsaric way of thinking, that's having a good time, but in fact, it is just confusion. Check it out with wisdom. Even though you say, "I had a great time," if you are honest, you will admit that it was just another old samsaric trip. We have had these experiences over countless lives, but our minds are still ignorant, uncontrolled, and undisciplined.

Therefore, don't be half-half. Cut off the wandering, confused mind by generating a strong, enthusiastic motivation: "I am extremely fortunate to have come to the conclusion, at least this once, that it is worthwhile to discipline my body, speech, and mind, and to have the opportunity of acting strongly to put myself on the path of perfect peace."

Then, when you take your seat before each session, you can think, "For the sake of all mother sentient beings, I must attain enlightenment on this very seat. I shall not move from it until I am one with Guru Heruka Vajrasattva."

Part 3

DISCOURSES

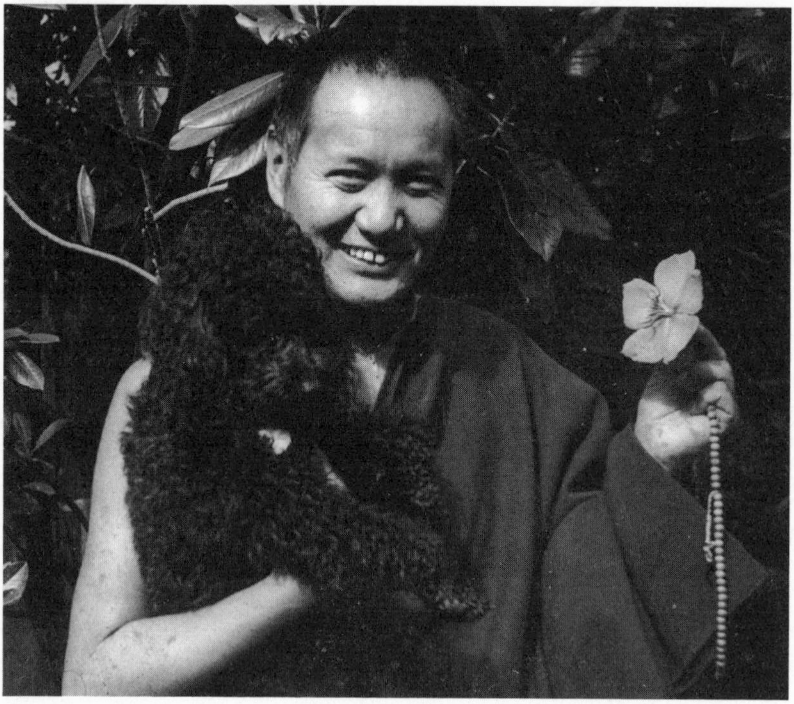

Photograph by Dorian Ribush

10

No Negativity Cannot be Completely Purified

THE MOMENT THE SUN RISES, the darkness of the night vanishes automatically. Similarly, when the light of wisdom appears in your mind, the dark shadow of ignorance naturally disappears.

Whenever you are depressed, anxious, or afraid, your view of the world becomes more distorted than ever, and your wrong conceptions multiply. Whenever your confused, dissatisfied mind arises, you become foggy and unclear. Even if you are outside in the sun or under a spotlight, there is darkness in your mind.

Therefore, it is highly beneficial to practice such a powerful tantric method as the yoga of Heruka Vajrasattva, which facilitates the growth of wisdom in your mind.

Most spiritual practitioners have taken vows and commitments as part of their religious practice. Those who lack wisdom feel that when they have broken some of their promises, they have done something irreversibly negative and become permanent sinners: "Oh, I promised not to do that, and now I've gone and broken my vow! Now I'll never be saved." That's a big misconception. All relative phenomena in the realm of the senses are impermanent, changing all the time. By their nature, they will cease of their own accord.

Another misconception is the depressed thought that you are hopeless. "Try as I might, I am always making mistakes." That's not true. Nobody is completely negative. We all have a positive side and a negative side.

In his Vajrayana teachings, the Buddha explained that although the root downfalls of tantra are the highest vows of all, even they can be restored when broken. Such transgressions are extremely negative, but since they are psychological phenomena, they can be purified.

In his Vinaya teachings, which are part of the Sutrayana path, the Buddha taught that there are certain unwholesome actions, such as murder, that cannot be fully purified in this lifetime. Thus, if you have broken one of the five precepts, you might feel that you have become permanently stained and get terribly upset. But you must remember that Lord Buddha gave his numerous different teachings according to the varying psychological needs of his many disciples. Sutra teachings were given to followers of a certain level of intelligence.

In the Vajrayana, the Buddha taught that there is no negativity that cannot be completely purified by the powerful methods of tantric yoga. Thus, you should never feel that because you have broken your vows or, for example, committed one of the so-called five inexpiable sins, you are a hopeless sinner beyond redemption.[18]

On the other hand, you should not rationalize that just because any negativity can be purified, you are free to do whatever you like. A broken cup can be repaired, but it's never the same as it was. Therefore, even though your vows and commitments can be restored when breached, it is better to keep them intact.

The best way to practice the Heruka Vajrasattva purification is in a three-month retreat, during which you recite the mantra one hundred thousand times. I usually ask students who want to take the Heruka Vajrasattva initiation to make a three-month retreat commitment. Also, it is easier for them to do this in the East than in the West, where the busy environment makes it almost impossible to find the time.

The retreat should be conducted under the right conditions, as explained in the retreat section of this book. Very few, if any, students have been able to follow these instructions to the letter. It is very difficult to adhere strictly to the ideal retreat discipline. Nonetheless, many conscientious and sincere Westerners have tried to do so, and although their concentration may not have been that strong, their three-month retreat has definitely changed their minds for the better.

Therefore, it is of great benefit to undertake this retreat, but make sure that the conditions you create are conducive to success. If I'm sitting here and someone is poking me with a needle, saying, "Come on, Lama, meditate, meditate," it's impossible. In the same way, it is hard to retreat in the middle of a city vibrating with the energy of aggression and desire. That's why Tibetan lamas always tried to find peaceful, isolated settings for their retreats. Good vibrations automatically help your practice.

If you can practice the Vajrasattva yoga method according to this commentary, there is no doubt that you will receive a most powerful purification. Why do you lack knowledge-wisdom and realizations? Because your mind is thickly clouded with the negative vibrations of delusion. The heavy obstacle of your ego concepts and an emotional inability to cope with problems allow no space. Wisdom cannot grow in this unclear atmosphere.

The Mahayana tradition emphasizes a combination of purifying and wisdom-generating meditations, rather than a preponderance of one over the other. When you purify the obscuring hindrances, your innate wisdom has a chance to develop. Thus, far from being contradictory, meditations on the graduated path and Vajrasattva purification are in complete harmony, and if you practice them together, you will quickly gain realizations.

Of course, I understand that not everyone is able to find the right circumstances for a three-month retreat at this time. Each of us has prior commitments and responsibilities according to his or her individual karma. If you can't commit yourself to the retreat, you shouldn't take the initiation and then feel as if you're somehow a prisoner of the Dharma. Lord Buddha's teachings are for freedom, not bondage! And those of you who cannot devote themselves to intensive practice should not feel inferior to those who can. You have to accept your present situation. The time will come when you will be able to find an ideal retreat situation. At that time you can take the Vajrasattva initiation with a three-month retreat commitment. Don't feel that you are unlucky or bad. It's not true. You are still very fortunate. You can maintain a daily practice on the graduated path to liberation, and do shorter retreats as time permits.

To develop your loving kindness, you can do Avalokiteshvara retreat. For wisdom, you can retreat on Manjushri. To overcome weakness and feelings of inadequacy, you can do Vajrapani retreat. There are many different retreats you can do according to your need. Retreats are like therapy. In the West, when you are sick you get therapy to cure your illness. Retreats are similar: you put yourself into a certain situation depending upon what the particular problem is. That's why I say that retreat is like medicine: an antidote to both the disease and its symptoms.

Why is purification so powerful? Because your wisdom and method are powerful. There is not some supreme power up in the sky washing your sins away. Power comes from your mental approach, the psychological key to the yoga method.

As I said before, the Heruka Vajrasattva tantric yoga method can purify the worst negativities you can imagine, including broken tantric, bodhisattva, and pratimoksha vows. It also purifies the symptoms of dissatisfaction, such as anxiety neuroses, inferiority complexes, and arrogant pride. Therefore, whenever you find you have broken your vows you should not get emotionally upset and feel hopeless and depressed. That's not wise. Instead, just be aware of what has happened, understand the interdependence of your uncontrolled negative mind and the conditions that caused you to break your vows, and skillfully apply the methods of purification.

You can learn a lot from such experiences. Analyze your mind. Intellectually, you do not want to do things that you have vowed not to do, but your uncontrolled mind interacts with the conditions and forces you to do them. Hence, you can understand your karma and see how powerful it is. You know from your studies on the graduated path that your precious human rebirth gives you the potential to do anything. How can you feel hopeless and depressed?

Do not belittle the teachings on the graduated path, thinking that they are too simple for you, the great practitioner of tantra. They are not at all simple but really most profound. This is not the hyperbole of a true believer but a scientific fact that you can prove for yourself by understanding and practicing the graduated path. In this way you can extract the essence from your precious human life, and instead of degenerating, you can progress. It is entirely in your own hands.

When you understand the graduated path clean-clear, you can see the benefits of purification retreat. At that time you are ready and qualified for such a retreat. If you don't know who or what you are, you can't practice even the graduated path properly, let alone the profound methods of tantric yoga.

Once you understand the nature of your life and the possibilities offered you by Dharma practice, you can choose your direction with wisdom instead of blindly following your ignorant wrong conceptions, as you've been doing for countless lives. You can choose your future because you now know how to create its causes. The past is finished, done with. What's the use of getting emotionally distraught over broken vows and other non-virtuous actions? You are not only wasting your time, but you are also piling negativity upon negativity. If, instead of applying the antidote when you recognize a non-virtue, you become emotionally disturbed, you are doubling your bad karma. You should be purifying your negativities, not becoming more sick.

Recently I read about a banker who committed suicide because he was caught embezzling funds. Was that the way out? He stole, felt guilty, got emotionally disturbed, and killed himself. That's a good example of what I'm saying: he has already created the negativity of stealing, but what are they going to do to him? Jail him, perhaps. Maybe confiscate his property. But they're not going to kill him, are they? Nevertheless, he couldn't bear the loss to his reputation, so he took his own life. We're the same. We do something negative then almost kill ourselves with guilt and worry. What's the use? It's completely self-destructive.

New experiences now lie ahead, and you can change direction to meet or avoid them as you choose. I'm not suggesting that you have the psychic power to see telepathically the details of your future, but I am saying that through analyzing your past experiences and drawing upon your understanding of the law of karma, you can deduce what you should and should not do. Checking in this way is very useful; worry is ridiculous.

Also, it is not enough to feel distress over and want to purify the horrible things you have done. As well, you should think that if you continue to do such things, you will only experience greater suffering in the future. Therefore, in addition to purifying past negative karma, you must also avoid creating actions motivated by ignorance, attachment, and anger. If you purify the non-virtuous actions you created in the past and refrain from creating them again, you can avoid the suffering result. The main factor that determines the kind of karma created by your actions is your motivation. It is up to you whether that motivation is positive or negative.

Although I was talking before about the negativity of breaking precepts, you should not feel that by taking precepts you have somehow imprisoned yourself. It's exactly the opposite. Precepts make you free. Some people feel a sense of loss after they have taken precepts. They feel a heavy weight upon their shoulders. If you understand precepts correctly, you will feel happy when you have taken them, because you know that you are well on your way to a blissful destination.

If your mind is limited, you will probably feel guilty or depressed when you break a precept. Say, for example, you have taken the eight Mahayana precepts for a day. During the morning ceremony you generated bodhicitta and the enthusiastic determination to keep the vows perfectly for the benefit of all sentient beings. But that evening somebody offers you a piece of chocolate. Unconsciously, out of habit, you eat it. Then you panic: "Oh my god! This morning I promised not to eat after midday, and now I've broken my vow. It's completely gone!" Many people react like this, but what's gone? There's no such thing as "completely gone." You kept the precept perfectly from the time you took it until you inadvertently broke it. You didn't break it intentionally. None of that positive energy has been lost.

Instead of beating up on yourself when you break a precept, you should rejoice: "Unbelievable! I really meant not to eat, but my old habits snuck up and cheated me when I wasn't looking." Feel happy about the time you kept the precept purely, and be happy to learn how your negative mind works. In this way your experience becomes wisdom. Taking precepts increases your awareness: it helps you understand karma at its deepest levels by bringing to your notice the subtle way in which it expresses itself. If you didn't take precepts, you would remain unaware of your negativities and would never know that they were there in your subconscious.

Without understanding this, you will never be really happy. You might take precepts but later regret it. "Oh, I made a mistake. I didn't realize it until I got back home to the West, but that Kopan lama must have hypnotized me!" Anyway, I'm joking, but some people might think along those lines. It is well worth taking precepts, even though you might break them occasionally. If you check up wisely, you will realize that you are really fortunate to take precepts. You don't break them on purpose, but you see how your old habits push you to break them unconsciously. That's a very useful revelation. That's how you develop your wisdom.

11

An Initiation Into Heruka Vajrasattva

The basic qualification for undertaking a tantric practice, such as the purifying yoga method of Heruka Vajrasattva, is a clear understanding of the three principal aspects of the path to enlightenment: renunciation, bodhicitta, and right view, sunyata. I'm sure you have a reasonable understanding of these, but day by day, year by year, you should be constantly striving to deepen it.

There are also many aspects to purification, such as making prostrations, reciting texts, and practicing the yoga methods of other deities. But the Heruka Vajrasattva method is perhaps the most powerful of all. This is just what we need. And while the Geluk tradition of Mahayana Buddhism stresses the great importance of purification, we need more than that. We have to integrate other activities—such as studying the teachings on the graduated path to enlightenment and helping others—into our practice of the purifying meditations of the yoga method. Some people seem to think that it's enough to practice only these meditations, but they're wrong. We have to take the middle way of balanced activities.

Old students who have done the three-month Vajrasattva retreat know just how profound a method of purification it is. New students will find out. It's not easy, but simply trying to face up to and overcome the difficulties is extremely worthwhile.

Now, as well as giving you a retreat commitment with this initiation, I'm going to add another condition. Based on my own experience of observing my students over a period of years, I have come to the conclusion that group retreats are much better for you than individual ones. In a way, that should be obvious. We all have a certain degree of knowledge-wisdom—don't think that knowledge is the exclusive domain of Tibetan lamas. Within each of us, certain aspects of it are better developed than others, so when we come together as a group, our collective wisdom forms a deep pool that we all can share.

For example, one day you might be feeling strong, but I'm overwhelmed by delusion. I can come to you and say, "Look, I'm freaking out here...what should I do?" You have the answer. This is what we mean by Sangha. You're having a hard time, you express your feelings to a Dharma brother or sister, and that person gives you wisdom, strength, and a solution to your problem. That's why I'm adding the condition of group retreat. I hope you understand. I'm not on a power trip: "This is *my* initiation; you have to do it my way." No! I just want this experience to be as beneficial for you as possible.

When we do Dharma things, we should do them professionally, with understanding. The Vajrasattva retreat has been structured to be of maximum benefit to the human mind, so you should do it properly. But having said that, I want to stress that you can retreat only to the best of your ability. In my commentary and retreat instructions, I'm a little bit strict, and it's true that strict is better. But if you can't practice exactly as I suggest, you shouldn't just give up altogether. You can't always do what you want to do, because you're subject to your own limitations. You have to accept yourself as you are and take it from there. Encourage yourself: "Well, it was a bit difficult today. I couldn't do the visualizations exactly as Lama recommended. But still, I got the main things right; I didn't break any sessions and did them as best I could. It was just that my concentration was a bit off."

I know that my Western students want to do things 100 percent as I say, and that's a beautiful quality. It's good to do anything perfectly. But you have to be reasonable. When you encounter difficulties, accept them. Sixty percent is better than nothing, better than running around the world like a wild animal with a confused mind. Think: "I may not be perfect, but I'm still better off trying to do the mantra as well as I can and giving energy to my Dharma brothers and sisters."

And if you can't do the meditations as explained, generate compassion instead. Remember the compassion that you feel for yourself when you're having a difficult time, and transfer that compassion to all mother sentient beings. Crying with compassion for others while reciting the Vajrasattva mantra is okay. It's certainly a lot better than just sitting there thinking, "I'm bad, I'm bad, I'm bad." Meditating with bodhicitta while reciting the Vajrasattva mantra is fine. As long as part of your mind is watching with mindful awareness that your mantra recitation is correct, you can generate compassion for others instead of doing the more complicated visualizations. I want new people to be clean-clear that this kind of skillful technique—directing whatever energy arises into the right channel—is permissible.

So, people who have done the retreat can take the initiation without having to do the retreat again. For new people, there's no consideration; you have to do the retreat. But when you do it, despite what I've been saying, I don't want you just to take it easy, mixing a little samsara with your nirvana. That doesn't work. Your retreat should be as pure a liberation, nirvana trip as you can make it. Our tendency is to mix things up—not this time, okay?

One thing that will make your retreat easier is being strongly dedicated to doing it well. If you're a bit wishy-washy about doing it—"maybe I should; maybe I shouldn't"—or if your mind is agitated, or you have a lot of expectations, then you can really freak out. You'll always feel like you're missing something: "Why am I sitting here? If I were in Melbourne I'd be having a good time. Why should I stay here?" This kind of question will arise. I would like you to be very single-minded about doing retreat—clean-clear and dedicated. Then you'll be comfortable: just sitting on your meditation cushion will be a blissful experience. And should superstitious thoughts bother you, remember the techniques for dealing with them, such as vase-breathing meditation explained in the commentary. Practice that, and when your mind is calm again, return to what you were doing.

I'd also like to add a point about mantra recitation to what I've already said in the main commentary, although perhaps I shouldn't state this publicly in case you start rationalizing. However, if after a couple of months' retreat you find you have very good single-pointed concentration, and you know from experience exactly how many mantras you recite in a session, you can recite the mantra silently, without using your rosary. But before you do this, be sure you have reached that level of development, and don't let your rationalizing mind cheat you.

Old students who have already done the retreat and completed their mantra commitment but would like to retreat again can do so alone, without joining a group. They can also practice mental recitation or even concentration without any recitation at all. After you have gone through the sadhana and become Vajrasattva, you concentrate on the blue seed syllable HUM at your heart and focus on that alone. You can work up to it by doing verbal recitation, then go deeper and deeper to mental recitation, and finally don't even do that but just concentrate single-pointedly on the seed syllable HUM. This can be very useful.

Now, before I give the initiation, I'm going to do a ritual to purify hindrances. These are subtle, formless manifestations of ego energy that prevent us from receiving the initiation perfectly and must be dispelled before we proceed. We transform this energy into some kind of wrathful form, and visualize Lama Heruka Vajrasattva chasing it away, beyond this solar system, from where it can never return. So, while I do the ritual, you meditate like that.

THE HERUKA VAJRASATTVA INITIATION

[Lama Yeshe gave the initiation stage-by-stage in the following, unique, way: first he explained the visualization to be done by the disciples; then he recited the text in English while the students did the visualization just explained; finally he recited the text in Tibetan. What follows below is the explanation, published in order to give readers an idea of the initiation process. Technically, this is not a full initiation (wang) *but is instead what is usually called "permission to practice"* (je-nang).*]*

The essence of Heruka Vajrasattva is the collected pure energy of all enlightened beings. This energy manifests as the white, blissful, radiant body of the deity. So when you take the initiation, instead of seeing the lama as a confused, ordinary person, transform him into the translucent appearance of the deity.

Then, according to tradition, you must ask him three times to confer the empowerment upon you. This is because we don't allow people the presumption of saying, "Hey! I've got a perfect, powerful, and very speedy method of attaining enlightenment. Come here, and I'll give it to you." Before they can receive an initiation, students have to be properly qualified and must request it most sincerely. So repeat three times after me: "Lama Vajrasattva, please give me the divine initiation of Vajrasattva."

Then you have to generate the enlightened attitude of bodhicitta. This is to ensure that your taking the initiation does not become a selfish power trip but instead an action dedicated to the enlightenment of all sentient beings. However, today you are not taking the full bodhisattva ordination of sixty-four vows but simply generating the strong motivation to use the yoga method for the sole purpose of benefiting others and not for any personal, temporal pleasure. With the divine, dedicated thought of reaching the highest destination—the everlasting, blissful realization of enlightenment—repeat three times after me: "The only reason I want to take this initiation is so that I can practice the yoga method in order to attain the everlasting, peaceful state of enlightenment for the benefit of other sentient beings."

Now remember, you receive the actual initiation only if your mind communicates, or meets together, with that of Lama Heruka Vajrasattva in the same space, or at the same level of consciousness. To generate that experience, it is very important that your concentration remain strong throughout the entire initiation.

From the seed syllable HUM at Lama Heruka Vajrasattva's heart, much powerful white radiant light comes into your heart, its electric energy magnetically burning your ego's conception, your image, of your entire physical nervous system, transforming it into white radiant light. This light dissolves and condenses, becoming smaller and smaller until it completely disappears into empty space. Concentrate on that emptiness.

Suddenly, in that empty space, a precious lotus flower appears. On the lotus flower appears a moon disc. At the center of the moon disc appears a radiant white vajra—the essence of your consciousness. Radiant white light emanates from the moon disc and vajra, embracing all of space. The all-embracing radiant light returns to sink into the vajra, the essence of your consciousness. The absorption of the light into the vajra acts as the cooperative cause for your consciousness to transform into the translucent, rainbow body of Heruka Vajrasattva—no flesh, no blood, no bone.

Your right hand holds a vajra, and your left hand holds a bell, signifying your complete realization of method and wisdom. You are embraced by the divine female, Nyem-ma Kar-mo, whose translucent holy body is also made of radiant white light and whose realizations are equal to yours, energizing within you the transcendental, blissful experience of the fully awakened mind.

You, Heruka Vajrasattva, are adorned with a radiant white OM at your crown chakra, a radiant red AH at your throat chakra, and a radiant blue HUM at your heart chakra.

From the white seed syllable OM and the Heruka Vajrasattva mantra that surrounds it at Lama Heruka Vajrasattva's crown chakra, powerful radiant white light emanates, pervading universal space and invoking all the supreme beings' pure energy, which transforms into blissful, radiant white light and sinks into the crown chakra of you, Heruka Vajrasattva. Like a powerful, rushing waterfall, this energy enters your Heruka Vajrasattva body, filling your nervous system with blissful, radiant white light, especially your crown chakra. That blissful experience purifies countless lives' accumulated impurities of body.

From the red seed syllable AH and the Heruka Vajrasattva mantra that surrounds it at Lama Heruka Vajrasattva's throat chakra, powerful radiant red light emanates, pervading universal space and invoking all the supreme beings' divine speech, which transforms into blissful, radiant red light and sinks into the throat chakra of you, Heruka Vajrasattva. Your Heruka Vajrasattva nervous system is completely filled with blissful, radiant red light, especially your throat chakra. That blissful experience purifies countless lives' accumulated impurities of speech.

From the blue seed syllable HUM and the Heruka Vajrasattva mantra that surrounds it at Lama Heruka Vajrasattva's heart chakra, powerful radiant blue light emanates, pervading universal space and invoking all the supreme beings' divine, transcendental wisdom, which transforms into blissful, radiant blue light and sinks into the heart chakra of you, Heruka Vajrasattva. Your Heruka Vajrasattva nervous system is completely filled with blissful, radiant blue light, especially your heart chakra. That blissful experience purifies countless lives' accumulated impurities of mind.

Now, simultaneously, from Lama Heruka Vajrasattva's crown chakra, comes blissful, radiant white light, which enters the crown chakra of you, Heruka Vajrasattva; from Lama Heruka Vajrasattva's throat chakra comes blissful, radiant red light, which enters your throat chakra; from Lama Heruka Vajrasattva's heart chakra comes blissful, radiant blue light, which enters your heart chakra. Through this, you and Lama Heruka Vajrasattva are indestructibly unified.

A duplicate mantra emanates from the mantra at Lama Heruka Vajrasattva's heart, leaves through his mouth and enters the mouth of you, Heruka Vajrasattva, and sinks into your heart. This happens three times. The first time it encircles the seed syllable HUM at your heart; the second time it dissolves into the original mantra there, increasing its power and strength; the third time it dissolves into it, making it indestructible, now and forever.

Visualize the mantra as a rosary of electrical energy. The mantra is like fire. Fire has the property of automatically burning anything that it touches. Similarly, the mantra's electrical wisdom energy automatically burns all the impurities of negative energy. Repeat the mantra after me three times. After the third, think that the blessings of Lama Heruka Vajrasattva have made it indestructible.

Now, from Lama Heruka Vajrasattva, a duplicate Heruka Vajrasattva emanates, coming to the crown of your head, descending through your shushuma, and entering your heart. Your body, speech, and mind are completely unified with Heruka Vajrasattva's divine body, speech, and mind.

Here, Tibetan lamas have a method to help those whose concentration is not strong. We touch the crown of your head with this torma that has the painting of the deity on top of it. As you file past and I touch you with it, concentrate strongly that Heruka Vajrasattva comes down your shushuma into your heart, and that the body, speech, and mind of you, Heruka Vajrasattva, are completely, non-dualistically unified with the divine body, speech, and mind of Heruka Vajrasattva.[19]

Now the initiation has finished. As you repeat the dedication prayers after me, make a heartfelt request for your group retreat to be as successful as possible.

You can see from your experience of this initiation that for the person whose concentration is very good, the process itself can be an enlightening experience. This highlights the difference between the Vajrayana and the Hinayana and Paramitayana schools of Buddhism. There, the emphasis is upon avoiding the kind of enjoyments that we grasp at; in tantra, we have the powerful wisdom and method to transform this ordinary energy into the blissful path to enlightenment.

This principle is not entirely dissimilar from the way modern scientific technology employs the earth's resources in an attempt to improve people's standard of living. Of course, the shortcomings of this approach are now becoming evident, with even politicians decrying the depletion of these resources and the pollution of our environment—something that can never happen through Dharma practice. When we take energy and, through skillful wisdom and method, transform it into the blissful path to enlightenment, no negative vibration can result.

It is most important that during your retreat you strongly maintain the transcendental experience that your entire consciousness has been transformed into the blissful, radiant white light body of Heruka Vajrasattva. You must really believe this. The psychological benefit of this is that you remove all thoughts of, "I am Thubten Yeshe; therefore, I'm hungry. I am Thubten Yeshe; therefore, I'm thirsty. I am Thubten Yeshe; therefore, I need beautiful objects." This eradicates your entire ego projection. It's incredible—the Mahayana has fantastically powerful methods of overcoming all your ego's vibrations. This is an extremely important part of your retreat.

Now, when I say that you should strongly believe that you are Vajrasattva, I don't mean that you should think that your physical body has changed. I know the kind of Western, pseudo-scientific argument you're going to make: "My body is made of flesh and bone. How can I transform it into light?" Well, you can indeed say that, but I'm going to reply that besides your physical body, you have a psychic body, the body of your subtle consciousness. It is your subtle conscious body that transforms into the white, radiant, translucent, rainbow-light body of the deity, and you generate divine pride on that.

Divine pride is very important. Let me tell you why. Normally, we think, "I'm negative. I'm *this*; therefore, I'm negative." Do you know what

I mean? I'm talking about the fact that you feel guilty, even when you're not. Even though you're not a religious person, you still feel guilty. Don't think that only religious people feel guilt. I've had enough experience with Westerners to know that they always feel guilty about something or other, even non-religious Westerners. Perhaps you think, "Oh, I only feel guilty because I'm trying to be a Buddhist. If I give up Dharma, I won't feel guilty any more." That's not the way to get rid of guilt. Even non-religious people feel guilt.

The way to abandon feelings of guilt and low self-esteem, such as "I'm bad; I'm negative," is to generate divine pride and thereby transform all your negative thoughts into blissful wisdom energy. With this technique you can deal with any situation that arises: take that energy and transform it into divine white radiant light and emanate as the deity. That's why I said "strongly" before—you have to really believe that you are Heruka Vajrasattva instead of "I'm Thubten Yeshe, born in Tibet, having this mother, that father, escaped...refugee...hungry." You have to overcome your ego trip. Whenever the mundane thought "I am" arises, mundane body, speech, and mind manifest immediately. The moment you generate divine pride and experience transcendental transformation, you eliminate all ordinary conceptions. And while it is essential to do this during your meditation sessions, of course, it is also necessary during the breaks. Instead of coming down when the session finishes, going to lunch, and allowing old habits to arise, looking at each other with lust or anger, maintain the energy of divine pride.

You can see how such method and wisdom can help you control your deluded energy. And you can see this through your own experience, not just my words. If I tell you too much about how tantra contains all these incredible methods, you'll just think, "Oh, he's so arrogant. He's just boasting about the power Tibetan lamas are supposed to have." It'll be too much for you. But if you check up for yourselves, you'll taste the benefits. And before you retreat, study the commentary well. Read it sentence by sentence, stopping to check and meditate on each one. If you are clean-clear about whatever you do, you'll be free of doubt and agitation and feel very comfortable. That is both important and necessary for your retreat to be successful.

If you start to experience difficulties during retreat, don't think, "I'm bad; I'm not a good retreater." Instead, simply ask yourself, "Why is my retreat not going well?" You have the answer: "It's because of my incredible delusions. And I'm not the only one. All my poor mother sentient beings are in this situation." Cherish others instead of yourself, and feel much compassion for all universal sentient beings. Instead of crying neurotically when you're having problems during a session, a perfect technique is to transform the energy of the mantra into compassion. Of course, emotional tears are not necessarily bad; crying can also be a blissful experience.

For example, the first time people discover sunyata, they're incredibly shaken and can completely space out. Inside, they experience a blissful shaking sensation; psychologically, they are transported way into space and then suddenly brought down. They almost doesn't know what's going on. Philosophically, this appears to be the very antithesis of the sunyata wisdom experience, which is supposed to be totally divorced from emotion. But the experience of an individual who actually discovers sunyata for the first time, can be completely different.

Like the close disciple of Lama Tsong Khapa, who initially experienced emptiness during a teaching on it, thought he'd disappeared, and grabbed at his lapel. Lama Tsong Khapa laughed, and said, "My disciple so-and-so has just found himself on his shirt!" He went on to explain that that's how the experience is supposed to be. So crying is not necessarily bad.

When difficulties arise, remember the reason: "All sentient beings, including myself, are in this situation. We are all objects of compassion." If you realize compassion during your retreat, what more could you ask? That's perfect. After retreat your actions will be imbued with loving kindness. It's possible. But be skillful, too; learn to relax during retreat, and be skillful in the way you relax. I don't mean that you should just lie about.

After retreat, do the simple fire puja of Dorje Khadro, which I explain briefly in the next chapter. There are many kinds of complex fire pujas in the Tibetan tradition, but this one is fine for us. You can even do it in everyday life, whenever you feel psychologically unwell, heavy, or impure. Just make a fire and do the Dorje Khadro puja with much meditation. It's like tum-mo meditation—it burns all your impurities.

Q: At the end of the sadhana, we meditate on ourselves as Heruka Vajrasattva. How do we concentrate on this?

A: This kind of concentration is very profound—much more profound than concentration on an external object, which, because it's easier, is what we usually do. Sometimes people experience heart pain or a rapid heartbeat when they do this meditation. This will happen if you are not relaxed or if you don't recognize the object of concentration as being in the nature of consciousness. When you are meditating on yourself as Vajrasattva and concentrating on the HUM at your heart, if you think of your body as physical, your heart may start to hurt; this is because your thinking is too concrete. It is extremely important to recognize your body as formless, as a psychic body. If I'm sitting here meditating and try to put a physical HUM where my heart is, there's be no room for it. The space is occupied. But if it's all in the nature of consciousness, anything is possible. Therefore, it is necessary to visualize the HUM as blissful, transcendental, and in the nature of consciousness.

Ordinarily, a deluded, grasping man might look at a beautiful woman and feel some kind of samsaric bliss. Similarly, the blue HUM at Vajrasattva's heart is a blissful, or bliss-generating, object. Whenever you visualize it, you feel blissful. This is an important point. As a result, you will have good single-pointed concentration. Why? Because the object of concentration itself—in this case the blue HUM—gives you a blissful experience. When you have a blissful experience, you feel satisfied; the hole in your psychological stomach is filled. When your psychological stomach is satisfied, you don't feel lonely or dissatisfied. When you are lonely, you are dissatisfied.

Monks and nuns often feel lonely...well, we all feel lonely. It's true. We have to know these things. It's necessary—this is Dharma. Perhaps you think I'm talking about dirty things, but we have to understand the dirty things in our lives in order to know what to clean. So why do we feel lonely and dissatisfied? Because we're looking for satisfaction—no blissful experiences, so our psychological stomachs are hungry. I'm sure you understand what I mean.

12

A Brief Commentary on the Vajrasattva Sadhana

Tibetan Buddhism considers the Vajrasattva practice very important. We call this teaching *Gel-kyen dig-drib jong-wa dor-je sem-päi tri.*

Gel-kyen means hindrance; *dig* means negativity, some kind of immoral action; and *drib* means obscuration. The difference between these last two is a little technical, but both are hindrances. For an action to become a negativity, there has to be a negative motivation, such as one of the three poisonous minds of ignorance, attachment, and hatred. An obscuration is not necessarily created with negative motivation. For example, the dull, sleepy, sluggish mind that stops you from developing single-pointed concentration is an obscuration, but there's not necessarily any negative motivation behind it. There are many levels of good and bad within the mind. Therefore, when we say that the Vajrasattva meditation is very powerful in eliminating negativities, we don't mean only immoral negative actions but any kind of hindrance.

For example, some of us take precepts. We make a vow before the Three Jewels of refuge—Buddha, Dharma, and Sangha—to do or not to do certain actions. When we make these vows, we are enthusiastically determined and quite confident that we shall be able to keep them purely. But then circumstances change, our internal wall crumbles, and we break a precept. Never mind; we can purify such breaks.

On the other hand, sometimes Western students come to me feeling very guilty, thinking that they have broken one vow or another, but when I ask them exactly how they broke the vow, I find that they have not broken it at all. They have a kind of concrete understanding, "I should never do this," when usually it is not the action itself that breaks the vow but the attitude, or motivation, behind it. Thus, even though whatever you did might appear to be contrary to your vows, if your motivation was not negative, you did not necessarily break it.

The most important thing for you to know is that no matter what sort of negative symptoms you have, all can be purified by the yoga method of Heruka Vajrasattva. Buddhism, especially tantra, asserts that you can purify any negativity whatsoever.

When we think about certain heavy negativities, it seems as if they are somehow permanent, unchangeable, impossible to purify. This idea of self-existent negativity is most dangerous. Fundamentally, all positive and negative phenomena are interdependent and changeable in nature. Certain Hindu philosophies hold that objects of the five senses are composed of permanent, unchangeable, self-existent atoms. Western scientists used to believe that too; some still may. Those are wrong conceptions.

It is important for you to know that we ourselves and all other phenomena, such as sense objects or qualities of positivity and negativity, are interdependent and changeable. Especially in the context of purification, you should be aware that symptoms of negativity, like desire, or anger, or whatever else you can think of, never stay the same. For example, you enter a certain environment, and all of a sudden your mind changes; you start shaking. That demonstrates the impermanent character of these emotions. They come, and they go. And not only can you solve the problems of negativity temporarily, but you can also eradicate them completely and forever.

I believe that people who practice purification are brave: "I can face and overcome any problem, any difficulty." Don't think that they are practicing purification because they're miserable. Many followers of Western religions accept the philosophy of permanent sin, and therefore they feel guilty. You have to avoid the heavy attitude thinking that it's impossible to overcome negativity. From the tantric point of view, the practitioner of purification is brave: "I can do it. Even though I've made mistakes, I am sure there's a solution to my problems." That's the right attitude; you are not afraid to admit your negativities. "Yes, that was negative; that was my uncontrolled mind." You accept it, but you don't feel hopeless. "I can change my mind. Anyway, it has been changing constantly ever since I was born. Now I can change it for the better." It is very important to know this—very important.

Now, besides bravely seeing the possibility of purifying any hindrance, you should also understand that you can purify the *imprints* that negative actions have left on your consciousness. In Tibetan, we call these *pag-cha.* Over countless lifetimes you have repeatedly created negative action after negative action, each of which has left an imprint on your mind. Even though an action may have finished, its imprint is still there and will cause you to do that action again. With the right wisdom, all negative imprints can be completely purified.

Where do hindrances come from? From the unskillful, polluted, dark, dualistic, egotistic mind. The way to overcome them is to practice the Heruka Vajrasattva yoga method again and again. This builds up, or reinforces, the transcendental, pure energy within you so that you come to see things non-dualistically, in their true nature of emptiness, or sunyata. According to tantra, when you see things more realistically, they no longer appear concrete but blissful. When an object becomes blissful, it becomes a deity; it appears in divine form.

Sometimes we see each other as ugly, don't we? Ugly things irritate us. That's the problem. When we see things more realistically—for instance, the deeper nature of other human beings—we are transformed. Happiness and bliss are energized within us. As a result, we see the qualities of the deity within other human beings. What are these qualities? Wisdom and compassion. What is a deity? Fully developed wisdom and compassion, the qualities of enlightenment. This applies to any deity whatsoever.

The Sadhana

Taking refuge and generating bodhicitta

We take refuge in Buddha, Dharma, and Sangha, the Sangha of the three Buddhist vehicles. That means you can no longer say, "I'm a Mahayanist; I don't take refuge in Hinayana arhats." We take refuge in Sangha without differentiation. We also take refuge in both dakas and dakinis. You can't say, "I'll take refuge in males, but not in females." We take refuge in all bodhisattvas. And you particularly take refuge in the person (*lob-pön*) who gave you the empowerment of Heruka Vajrasattva.

The principal object of refuge is standing two-armed Heruka, holding a vajra and bell, embracing his consort Vajravarahi. It might be too difficult for you to visualize the aspect with all the arms and legs. They are surrounded by all the figures mentioned in the main commentary, who fill all of space. These melt into light and dissolve into Heruka, who then sinks into you. You become Heruka. Concentrate on that for as long as you can.[20]

When you generate bodhicitta by thinking, "I must become Heruka...," you can send radiant light into the ten directions, purifying all sentient beings in the six realms and transforming them into Heruka. All these Herukas then sink into you. That is one technique for actualizing bodhicitta.

The actual yoga method

When doing the Heruka Vajrasattva yoga method, you can visualize yourself as Heruka, or Vajrapani, or whomever else is your favorite deity. But then the question might arise, "If I am Heruka, what need is there to purify?" Of course, if you really are Heruka you certainly don't need any purification. Here, when you transform yourself into the divine aspect of Heruka, even if you have very good concentration, your dualistic mind will be lurking somewhere in the depths of your consciousness, just waiting to jump out and confuse you.

This reminds me of a story about a Yamantaka practitioner in Tibet. As you know, Yamantaka has all these hands, each one holding something or other. One day this monk was visualizing himself in that aspect, and he must have been quite convinced, because when his lama tried to give him something, he said, "Sorry, my hands are full." So his lama replied, "Well, just use your regular, impure hands instead."

Even if you can visualize yourself as Heruka with complete conviction, not an ordinary thought in mind, you still need purification. Not just because Buddha says so, but because your dualistic mind is still there. Therefore, even if you manifest as Heruka, you can still practice the Heruka Vajrasattva method. When you do, however, you simply maintain divine appearance without emphasizing divine pride.

Visualize Heruka Vajrasattva above your crown, at whatever height is comfortable for you. However, he shouldn't be miles above you—a hand's breadth, or something like that is enough. His body is not like our material, physical bodies but is a rainbow body: clear and transparent, a psychic body. He is completely unified with his consort. She symbolizes enlightened wisdom; he, enlightened method.

Light radiates from his heart into the ten directions, invoking all the buddhas and bodhisattvas. This white radiant light is the energy of divine, enlightened wisdom, the pure knowledge-wisdom that understands the deepest nature of totality. That is the pure mind. The impure mind is just the opposite. It is narrow; it lacks skillful wisdom and produces impure actions.

The white radiant light of supreme wisdom-energy that is invoked sinks into Heruka Vajrasattva's heart, goes down his shushuma to his secret chakra, into Dorje Nyem-ma's secret chakra, and fills her shushuma, too. Their bodies are filled with blissful white radiant light. From the mantra at the heart of each deity, blissful white kundalini energy rushes down their central channels, through their secret chakras and into your crown chakra. It is very powerful, like a waterfall. In this yän-de visualization, white light rushes down your shushuma pushing out through your secret chakra all negative energy and impurities in the aspect of pigs, chickens, snakes, and so forth. These and other animals, like scorpions, monkeys, and cows, symbolize all the different sorts of negativity within your nervous system. All are completely flushed out. Your dissatisfaction and loneliness are also purified, as are any other disturbing negative symptoms that you can think of.

You can also do män-de visualization at this point. Here, you visualize all your internal garbage floating up on the surface of the blissful kundalini energy as it fills your body from bottom to top. This garbage leaves your body through your nose, eyes, mouth, and ears, and also bubbles out your crown chakra.

Then you can do the third meditation, or phung-de, visualizing brilliant radiant light. It beams down from Vajrasattva's heart, through his secret chakra and then through your crown, and purifies your entire nervous system. These are the three visualizations to do while you are reciting the mantra.

At the end, Heruka Vajrasattva sinks through your shushuma into your heart. Your body, speech, and mind are unified with his divine body, speech, and mind. You become Heruka Vajrasattva. From your divine heart much light radiates through the six samsaric realms, purifying all sentient beings and transforming them all into the aspect of Heruka Vajrasattva. All these Heruka Vajrasattvas then sink into you.

This is important. We are always involved with other people and often have heavy karma with each other. We get angry with others; we get strongly attached to others. Most of our problems are with other people. We are so strongly connected that we go through our entire lives constantly bumping into each other.

When you do the above meditation, you transform yourself, and you also transform all objects. Thus, for you there are neither objects of craving desire nor objects of hatred, so you remain healthy. The Vajrayana places great emphasis on the transformation of objects so that rather than energizing the three poisons of ignorance, attachment, and anger within you, they energize bliss instead.

You also emit from your divine Heruka Vajrasattva heart countless manifestations of Heruka Vajrasattva and whatever else you consider attractive and desirable—beautiful men, beautiful women, or any other beautiful object of the senses—as offerings to the supreme beings in the ten directions. Visualize that this offering gives great bliss to those buddhas and bodhisattvas. In fact, the essential meaning of the word "offering" is that which energizes transcendental bliss in whomever receives it. That is a proper offering. If you give something that causes suffering, it's not an offering. Since the Buddhist connotation of offering is that which brings happiness, you can see that most of the time our gifts don't work that way; even though we mean well, our presents often make people miserable.

So much for the essential points of the sadhana. You now have to understand the actual purpose of the transformation we are practicing here. If someone asks you why you are practicing this yoga method, you might reply, "To purify myself." Well, that's basically okay, but the real answer should be, "I want to understand the true nature of all existence; I want to understand reality." That's the real purpose of the Heruka Vajrasattva yoga method. It shows you what is reality and what is not; it helps you realize sunyata, non-duality, and stops you from continuing under the influence of the concrete conceptions of your ego.

The more you understand the fundamental nature of all existence, the greater the bliss you experience. The greater the bliss you experience, the closer you are to attaining the beautiful form of the deity. That is the main point.

Many Westerners think that it must be painful to understand samsara the way it's explained in Buddhism: "Buddhism says that life is suffering; that means there's no way out!" It seems that Buddhist philosophy and meditation were created for the express purpose of making people miserable! That's a completely wrong attitude; they don't understand what they really need.

What I'm saying is that the whole purpose of practicing Heruka Vajrasattva is to realize non-duality—the fundamental reality of yourself and all other phenomena. That realization is an extremely blissful experience. Once you've experienced that bliss, you can see the beauty of the deity in every other person and stop putting negative projections onto others.

Tantric philosophy teaches that whoever practices tantra must see other sentient beings as deities. That's the *philosophy*. Those who have realized the fundamental nature, the non-duality, of other human beings have the transcendental experience of seeing the enlightened qualities of the deity in others. Such practitioners have no room for negative thoughts.

Those are the main points; I hope it's enough. Are there any questions?

QUESTIONS AND ANSWERS

Q: We are supposed to see others as Heruka Vajrasattva, but what happens when we see someone doing something negative?

A: You mean, should you try to stop them? Well, remember the story about the monk who was visualizing himself as Yamantaka? It's similar. If you see someone doing something wrong, you can say, "Hey, what's going on?" The thing is, however, that you still have to see Heruka Vajrasattva somewhere within him. It's just that he's forgotten who he really is and is acting under the influence of his chicken or snake mind. So you can say, "Excuse me, your chicken is showing!" Something like that!

My experience is that it's difficult to visualize women as, say, the male deities Vajrasattva or Vajrapani. But I try to see that somewhere within the atmosphere of the female body is the crystal, clean-clear psychic body of Vajrasattva or Vajrapani. You can understand that. Each of us does have Vajrasattva quality, Vajrapani quality within us, so we can visualize the divine body co-existing with us.

Q: Sometimes when I meditate I see a kind of blue light in front of me. Is it real or imaginary, and what does it mean?

A: It depends a bit on how you feel when you see it—whether you feel relaxed or irritated. But it's not necessarily just a mental projection. Sometimes when your mind has developed in a certain way, you can see light physically, with your eye sense. I think it's very good if someone has this kind of natural vision of light. Normally, when we meditate we don't see any light at all; only darkness. If I see green or blue light, even in my imagination, I feel happy. Blue light is somehow related to infinity; seeing blue light suggests a mind that's very expansive, not narrow.

Q: How big should you visualize Vajrasattva?

A: It varies with the person. Some people like to visualize him big, others small. He shouldn't be too big; most people tend to favor something similar to their own proportions. Also, he should not be heavy or physical, and he shouldn't touch your head. You don't have to force the visualization, either. He simply manifests in the space above your head, appearing spontaneously. Out of Heruka Vajrasattva's divine omnipresent wisdom his energy appears without effort, like a reflection in a mirror. If you don't have some understanding of sunyata, then he seems really heavy: "Oh, Vajrasattva is too heavy for me. This retreat's too heavy, and he's too heavy!" That shows you don't really understand the wisdom of non-duality.

Anyway, visualize Vajrasattva as whatever size feels comfortable but clean-clear, crystal, like a rainbow, so that just looking at him energizes a clean, blissful kundalini experience. Sometimes these experiences can feel like an orgasm, but they are not physical reactions. If you are meditating with intensive awareness, there's no problem, but if you don't have some understanding of non-duality, then things become too physical and that can be dangerous.

Q: Please would you say something about the quality of Heruka Vajrasattva.

A: Heruka Vajrasattva is the fully developed pure wisdom of the three time buddhas and bodhisattvas manifesting in a pure emanation of white radiant light. Therefore, his essence is non-dual wisdom. Whenever you practice the yoga method, his divine form is demonstrating reality for you. He is the eternally blissful state of pure wisdom.

Q: What does Heruka mean, and how is Heruka Vajrasattva different from other Vajrasattvas?

A: Literally, "Heruka" means drinking blood, but it symbolizes experiencing eternal bliss. Bliss has the quality of the totally developed unity of male-female energy. Dorje Nyem-ma holds a kapala containing what seems to be blood. That symbolizes her giving eternal blissful energy. When you practice Heruka Vajrasattva, you drink the blood of the emotion of the experience of eternal bliss. Red signifies emotion. As human beings we need to express emotion to each other. Some people are completely unemotional—they are just like wood. That's no good. Even if you are an enlightened being or in deep samadhi, you can still show emotion; it's just that you don't get involved in emotionally suffocating situations.

Heruka Vajrasattva has a kind of unique energy and emphasizes the development of wisdom. There are four classes of tantra; Heruka Vajrasattva is from the maha-anuttara yoga, or highest, class.

Q: When visualizing the two deities in union, do you visualize yourself as the male, the female, or both conjoined?

A: Whatever feels comfortable for you is good. As I said before, sometimes women find it difficult to visualize themselves as male deities and vice versa. But we all have male and female energy within us. Sometimes it gets unbalanced. Some men are too feminine, others, too masculine. The same goes for women. We have to develop the totality of the male-female energy that lies within each of us.

Also, when you look at Vajrasattva in union with his consort Dorje Nyem-ma, you cannot say that one is higher and the other is lower. They are both at the same level, totally unified in nature. If it's easier for you, you can visualize yourself as Yum Dorje Nyem-ma Karmo, with the Heruka Vajrasattva mantra at your heart. But no matter how you visualize the deity, the key is to visualize with intensive awareness of the fundamental nature of non-duality. If you do not, there's a danger that your visualization will become physical and will energize sense desire. The purpose of this practice is to eliminate desire.

Q: How far above your head can you visualize the deity? I find it easier to get a waterfall effect with the purifying energy when it's higher than the usual few fingers' breadth.

A: If it's easier, you can make it a little bit higher. Then, a tube of rainbow light emanates from his heart and connects with your crown chakra, and the blissful kundalini energy rushes down that.

Q: How can we use the Vajrasattva meditation to deal with feelings of guilt that might come up during the day?

A: Whenever you feel guilt arising, transform it into Heruka Vajrasattva. From head to toe, you are Heruka Vajrasattva. Also, besides the psychological effects of negative emotions, there are subtle physical effects that energize dissatisfaction. When you feel the energy of guilt within you, transform its subtle physical aspect into the Heruka Vajrasattva mantra. In that way it becomes the solution to your problems.

We need such active solutions to the negative habits that plague us. Knowing intellectually that they are negative is not enough to stop them. Here, we are acting in a practical way, building a defense against them instead of just dreaming. This is integrating Dharma with your daily life.

Retreat

When you retreat, you shouldn't push yourself too much. Sometimes retreat can feel quite heavy; three months can seem like an eternity. Also, Westerners often don't know how to retreat. I have given the technical details elsewhere, but as far your as attitude is concerned, you should think that the pleasure of retreat is like that of a nightclub. You're gaining blissful wisdom—enjoy yourself!

Take it easy. Make a schedule. If a session is difficult, not coming together, the techniques are difficult to master, the vase breathing too hard to do, take a break. Go outside. People feel, "Oh, retreat. I should be strict; I should be mean; I should struggle; I should give myself a hard time." It's not like that. Don't push.

You should keep yourself clean; wash regularly. And eat nutritious food. Don't try to be this big ascetic. Tibetan Buddhism teaches you to use all your energy—wealth, beauty, whatever—to bring yourself closer to enlightenment. That's what life is for.

The reason I mention all this is that Western people seem to think that retreat means not eating good food, not eating chocolate. That's stupid. Eat well—you're working for enlightenment. Don't treat yourself like a cow. Encourage yourself. I have to tell you that retreats have been the most pleasurable experiences of my life. I really enjoy them. I'm not hard line. Last time, at Tushita in Dharamsala, I had a hammock! In the breaks I'd go out and lie in it. The students used to gather round and look at me: "That's the way to retreat?" They couldn't believe it!

Retreats are for enjoyment, but not in the confused, samsaric sense of the word. There is something healthy to be gained; some satisfaction, some integration. Don't make your retreats unnecessarily difficult.

Fire puja

When you have finished your retreat, you should do the Dorje Khadro fire puja. This is very useful. It's a bit like tum-mo meditation.

You visualize at your heart a black seed syllable that draws into you all the sickness, disease, and other negative symptoms of yourself and all other sentient beings. At your navel chakra there's a fire. Wind energy comes up from your feet and fans the blaze until it's roaring like a furnace. The fire gets stronger and stronger and explodes up your shushuma, pushing all the negative energy from the black seed syllable at your heart out through your nostrils into the mouth of the deity. That is the basic meditation technique.

The actual fire burning in front of you activates your mind so that the meditation becomes more intensive and realistic, and that helps you to realize sunyata. This is the main point of the Dorje Khadro fire puja. There's no commitment to do this after the Vajrasattva retreat, but if you could do 110,000 or 115,000 Dorje Khadro mantras it would be very powerful and beneficial.

Do four meditation sessions a day. Before breakfast, you should do a Vajrasattva retreat session, but since you've already finished your mantra commitment, use the session for contemplation instead. By reciting all those mantras in retreat, you have already built up within you a certain essential energy—the "nuclear energy" of the mantra. So now, simply contemplate.

After breakfast, make the fire and do a two-hour Dorje Khadro session. Then have lunch, and after that have a rest, and study some Dharma books. In the late afternoon do another two-hour session of fire puja. Finally, in the evening, do another session of single-pointed concentration, again without verbal recitation of the Vajrasattva mantra.

Actually, you can do the Dorje Khadro fire puja any time you feel bothered, hassled, irritated, or uncomfortable. You don't have to be in retreat. Morning, afternoon, or night—it's very powerful, very useful. It can stop those feelings right there. This comes from Lama Tsong Khapa's experience; it was one of his favorite meditations. When you do it, you're getting a real taste of his practice. It's like gold, a real golden Dharma.

Sometimes we need to do these active meditations. Visualize Dorje Khadro, a manifestation of Guhyasamaja, with his huge gaping mouth open, like a powerful black hole, sucking everything into it. All negative energy disappears into it forever.

13

Vajrasattva Practice and Highest Yoga Tantra

Before you can practice the completion stage of maha-anuttara yoga tantra, among other things, such as guru yoga, you must practice the Vajrasattva yoga method.

The Panchen Lama said that in order to understand the reality of your mind, you have to do intensive purification and collect a vast amount of merit. Both are important.

Take, for example, our own experience. We are very enthusiastic and really want from the bottom of our hearts to enjoy deep meditation, but no matter how hard we try, we always encounter mental garbage, distractions, and the sluggish, sleepy mind. Without control, millions of concepts, negative thoughts, and superstitions gallop through our minds. That means something's missing. And what is that? Purification. We need a lot of purification.

You can't blame the practices you've been doing: "I've been meditating for two years, and I still haven't achieved single-pointed concentration. What's the point of meditating?" You can't say that. Every day your superstitious mind takes you on an unbelievable trip. In one night it can take you around the whole world. Every trip leaves deep karmic imprints in your mind. It takes a long time to eradicate these. So you shouldn't be arrogant: "I'm not particularly negative. I'm pretty pure. I've never killed anyone; I don't lie; my parents take care of me, so I don't have to fight and cheat for food and clothing. I don't need purification." That's just an ego trip.

Impurity comes from the mind as well as the body. Check out the trips that your mind has been on from the time you were born until now. It's unbelievable. If you look at those experiences in the light of the twelve links of dependent arising, you'll practically drown in the ocean of superstition. That's why we need a great deal of purification.

For example, it would be pretty hard to grow fine, delicate lettuce here in Dharamsala. The soil here is very rocky, and the weeds are out of control. The ground would need a lot of work. Similarly, our minds need a lot of purification to eradicate the gross superstitions that prevent our fine, most subtle consciousness from functioning.

Also, sometimes we might think we're very capable of doing something, but deep inside, a subconscious voice keeps saying, "I'm incapable, I'm incapable; I'm not good at anything. I'll never be liberated, never be enlightened, never be Vajrayogini." Inside, that kind of stuff is going on all the time. Within your subconscious, a million chickens are clucking, "Not possible, not possible"; a million snakes are hissing, "Not possible, not possible"; a million pigs are grunting, "Not possible, not possible." Your subconscious mind is deeply contaminated by billions of delusions like these.

You'd be surprised at how pervasive this contamination is. You truly believe at the intellectual level that "I can do it," but deeply concealed, the billion voices of the pig-snake-chicken "can't-do" mentality keep telling you that you can't.

It's a psychological thing. You might accept something intellectually—"I want to become Vajrayogini"—but simultaneously that voice keeps saying, "No, you don't." There is acceptance and rejection at the same time. You can't understand it. You get really confused: "Do I want it, or don't I? Do I want an apple or not?" You're not sure, not sure, not sure.

That's the dualistic mind. We always talk about the dualistic mind—that's it; that's how it works. The dualistic mind is always comparing two things. You want to achieve deep concentration and discover eternal liberation but at the same time you resist, you reject it. The human mind is very funny.

So you can see from the practical point of view that you do, in fact, need purification, because when you meditate there are so many hindrances. That is the logic, and it is based on your own experience. You definitely need purification. You can't say, "I'm meditating, that's enough." It's never enough. There's a clear difference between meditation and purification. As Manjushri told Lama Je Tsong Khapa, "Meditation is not enough. You also have to purify the hindrances and accumulate great merit. It is very important that these things be done simultaneously."

Now you can see why Manjushri advised Lama Je Tsong Khapa in this way: "Don't just meditate all the time. Do some purification, too." That also shows that Lama Je Tsong Khapa liked to meditate a lot. Many Western scholars think that Lama Je Tsong Khapa was just an intellectual —some sort of Tibetan Buddhist professor, not a meditator. But then Manjushri told him, "You are doing too much meditation. That's not enough. You also have to do purification and accumulate more merit." Lama Je Tsong Khapa was an unbelievable yogi. You cannot imagine. Even as a ten-year-old boy he was a great meditator. And when he was doing Manjushri meditation in retreat, a figure of Manjushri appeared spontaneously on the wall of his cave. I think you can still see that in Tibet.

Purification is very important. It is the only way to get rid of those billions of subconscious animals that keep telling you, "Not possible, not possible."

There's another slightly different psychological symptom, too: "It's not possible to purify, not possible to improve yourself, not possible to eradicate your dissatisfaction, not possible to release your attachment and desire." Does this sound funny? Check it out. At one level you want to do these things, but when you try, there's a voice deep down saying, "Hey, come on. It's not possible." That's what we call Mara, and he's there all the time.

This is why we don't have strong energy to purify ourselves, why we are not really convinced that we can overcome our grasping Western karma and gravitational attachment to sense pleasures. Go deep into your unconscious mind and you'll see what I'm talking about. Intellectually we know we can get enlightened, but deep down there's the hindrance that just keeps on saying, "No."

The point is this: the voice that tells you it's not possible to purify your negative karma also results from a lack of purification. That's the main point. In Buddhism we talk a lot about purification. We're talking about purifying the mind, not the body; purifying negative attitudes, negative psychological expressions. That's why it is extremely important to be totally convinced that you can purify any negativity whatsoever, any negativity you can think of. For example, Hitler exterminated millions of people. Even the murder of so many people can be completely purified, leaving not the slightest trace of negativity.

In Nagarjuna's *Letter to a Friend*, he tells the true story of Lord Buddha's brother, who had incredibly strong desire, more than all of ours put together. Still, he was able to purify that and become an arhat.

Then there was Angulimala, who followed the wrong guru and was told that he would not gain realizations until he had killed a thousand people. Believing this, he started killing people and had killed 999 when the Buddha appeared and showed him how wrong it was. Even he was able to purify his negativities and become an arhat. Finally, there was King Ajatashatru, who lived at the time of Lord Buddha. He committed one of the five inexpiable sins by imprisoning his father, who died in jail. Even this extremely negative karma could be purified, and he too became an arhat.[21]

Therefore, through these examples, you should understand that any negative karma that you have created in this life has been made by your pathetic, weak, illogical, grasping negative mind. The inner nuclear missile of your powerful, transcendental, simultaneously born great wisdom can definitely purify it all. You should be thoroughly convinced of this, not "Maybe it can, maybe it can't." Think instead, "It is 100 percent certain that any negativity I have created by body, speech, or mind can be completely purified." This brave, understanding mind is very, very useful. Without it you will never succeed in meditation, because those billions of animals in your subconscious will be telling you, "No, no, no, no, no, no, no...."

If you recite the Vajrasattva mantra twenty-one times every night, it stops the otherwise exponential proliferation of negative actions created during that day. Without purification, one day's negative energy will have doubled by the next, redoubled by the day after that, and so on. The tantric texts also explain that if you recite the mantra properly one hundred thousand times, you can completely purify all negativities whatsoever, even broken root tantric vows. There is no negativity that cannot be purified by this method. It's very powerful.

Also, as I've explained before, there are various aspects of Vajrasattva: kriya, charya, yoga, and maha-anuttara yoga. The latter also include the Guhyasamaja and Yamantaka aspects, which, as His Holiness Song Rinpoche said, emphasize physical purification, purification of the body. Heruka Vajrasattva focuses more on mental purification. That's why it is such a powerful method. Not only for Tibetans. It is possible that some practices that are suitable for Tibetans might not suit Westerners, but this is not one of them. I've been doing some anthropological experiments on my Western students, and so far I think that their Vajrasattva practice has been pretty successful. After retreat their brain is something else! I wasn't expecting such a big change. For some reason, practicing Heruka Vajrasattva transforms them into quite different human beings. I'm glad that Westerners find this practice so suitable and helpful.

The actual practice of Vajrasattva is quite simple. First, as I stressed before, you have to be aware of your negativities. You may not seem to have anything gross or anything that you're even aware of, but you certainly will have a lot of stuff deep down in your subconscious. When you practice the Vajrasattva meditation, you have to purify all these things. You also have to have strong confidence that you're capable of being purified, the strong belief that purification is possible, and the powerful determination never to repeat those negative actions ever again. The latter is one of the four opponent powers, which I have explained in the main commentary. Using those powers is the right way to purify.

The meditation itself is simple. I'll run through it very briefly. A few fingers' breadth above the crown of your head is a lotus and moon seat, upon which is a white vajra with the syllable HUM at its center. Light radiates in all directions purifying all mother sentient beings' environments and wrong conceptions; it then returns, unifying with and transforming the vajra into the radiant white body of Heruka Vajrasattva. Lama Je Pabongka describes different shades of white for the various aspects of Vajrasattva's body. The body itself is clear like crystal, the lotus at his heart is milky in color, the mantra around its edge is silver. Everything is still white, but differentiated slightly in order to help you visualize.

He has one face and two arms and holds a vajra in his right hand and a bell in his left. He embraces his consort, Dorje Nyem-ma, who holds a curved knife in her right hand and a kapala full of blissful energy in her left. Then blissful white kundalini energy gushes down from their hearts, through their shushumas to where they are joined at the lower chakra, through the lotus and moon seat, through your crown chakra, and down your shushuma, purifying all the conscious and unconscious negativities we were talking about before. And to do this, we use three different meditation techniques—män-de, yän-de, and phung-de—which I have described in detail elsewhere.

The great yogi Lama Je Pabongka further said that if you are doing completion stage practice, you can do a further visualization that will help you with it. When the blissful kundalini energy rushes down your shushuma, it energizes the four types of bliss—bliss, great bliss, extraordinary bliss, and extremely great bliss—as it passes through your crown, throat, heart, and navel chakras, respectively.

Also, when you think about negativity, don't just think physically, but purify mental weaknesses as well, such as sadness, loneliness, and so forth. Other benefits of the blissful energy pouring down your shushuma are that it helps you to open all your chakras and to develop tum-mo meditation and great bliss. So now you see that you can practice the Vajrasattva meditation at the simple level of the generation stage or the more advanced level of the completion stage.

Because the Vajrasattva practice allows you to overcome any sort of negativity, you become very courageous and liberated. You feel confident that anything is possible, that you can conquer any difficulty. That aspect is very important. It gives you great inspiration. The weak mind keeps saying, "Not possible, not possible, I can't do it, I can't do it, I can't decide, I can't decide." Some people can't even decide whether or not to go to the bathroom. What do you think of them? They need Vajrasattva meditation! It's true, unbelievable. I don't understand some people's minds. They can't decide about anything. My goodness. When I see people like that, I feel maybe I'm not so bad after all!

Purification is very useful. It gives you great satisfaction and flexibility of mind. You know you can do something. You can go into darkness; you can go into light; you can even go underground! You become confident in your ability to do anything.

I really hope that all my students will do at least one hundred thousand Vajrasattva mantras before they die. I truly believe that after doing a Vajrasattva retreat they cannot be reborn in the hell realms. No way! They can make a decision: "After the Vajrasattva retreat there's no way I can be reborn in a miserable realm. I don't care whether I live or die." You get some sort of insurance. Vajrasattva retreat is insurance against being reborn in the lower realms. We need such insurance. Now I'm becoming an insurance salesman! That's terrible, isn't it! Still, I need your help to make my insurance company successful.

Whether we are believers or non-believers, we do need some confidence. We're all impermanent. We don't know when we're going to die. We have all these shortcomings. But if you have indestructible insurance, who worries about death? Death is natural; worrying about it is a waste of time. Instead of feeling upset that your body is not as beautiful as it once was, look forward to being reborn with a better one. Anyway, I'm joking. My point is, however, that you need some kind of self-confidence, "I'm definitely going to die, but at least I'm guaranteed of not being reborn in the lower realms." There *is* such a guarantee, because there definitely exists a level of mind that you can reach, from which you cannot descend to a lower rebirth.

For those who cannot do the long mantra as a daily practice, His Holiness Song Rinpoche said that you can recite the short one: OM VAJRASATTVA HUM twenty-one times, before you go to sleep at night. It only takes a minute or two; anybody can do that.

Now, I want to make sure you understand clean-clear that you don't have to have killed, stolen, or beaten people up to need Vajrasattva purification. There's a deeper reason than just wanting to purify what people commonly refer to as negativity. What is negativity? Most people will interpret it as doing bad things to other people. Americans always say, "We didn't do bad things; we always help other people." That's a joke! They're fooling themselves. Even if you have devoted your entire life to helping others, the weak mind is still there. That's why you need purification.

One thing I have observed is that someone who has done very bad things is also capable of tremendous good. This may not be a fact, it's just something I've observed. Some people are almost numb. Neither their positive nor their negative actions have any strength; all their actions are like water. People like that tend to think, "I haven't done anything bad, I'm always careful. I don't need purification." They might be careful, but it's out of self-pity and concern for their own well-being. That doesn't mean they do not need purification.

Take Milarepa, for example. After his father died, the villagers confiscated his mother's property, so she sent Milarepa to a black magician to learn the craft so that later they could take revenge. One night all the villagers came together at somebody's house for a party. With his black magic Milarepa made the roof collapse, killing them all. You can see how he had built up a tremendous force of negative energy. He studied for years and then watched and waited for the right opportunity with only the negative motivation of killing all those people in mind. But later he was able to generate even more powerful positive energy, purify all this negativity, and reach enlightenment in that lifetime. In contrast, some people are ineffective either positively or negatively, completely wishy-washy.

Human potential is incredible. You can do such positive things. Jesus was unbelievably powerful. People thought he was crazy. Shakyamuni Buddha, too. He had enormous wealth and power, but he gave it all up, escaped from samsara, and became enlightened. People thought he was stupid: "If he'd remained as king, he could have done so much for others, but he went into the jungle to live like an animal. He's ridiculous." Humans have tremendous power and potential and can purify vast amounts of negativity.

If you want to practice the completion stage of tantra, you should first do one hundred thousand Vajrasattva mantras. Purification is important, because freedom from the dualistic mind *is* enlightenment. We talk about enlightened realizations, buddhahood. That's freedom from the dualistic mind. Purification eradicates the dualistic mind.

When Atisha was making the long overland trip from India to Tibet more than a thousand years ago, he kept stopping the caravan and jumping down to do purification at the side of the road. Whenever he noticed the slightest negative thought or concept, he would purify it then and there. That shows he was a great yogi, a great bodhisattva. That shows he understood karma. We don't understand karma; we just let it go. But he understood how negative karma multiplies in the mind, and so he made a point to purify it right away.

It depends on how sensitive you are. If you are sensitive, you notice the effect of even the slightest negative karma. If you are immersed in an ocean of negative karma, you don't feel it. The heavy blanket of negativity is always there.

Once there was a great lama who was so pure that he always had a vision of light in front of him. One day a Tibetan family invited him to do a puja at their house. But the money they had used to buy the food and tea they offered him had come from the sale of *prajñaparamita* texts, books on the perfection of wisdom. As you know, money from the sale of holy objects like books and statues should not be used to buy temporal needs.

When the lama got home that night he noticed that his vision of light had disappeared. That was because he had eaten impure food that day. If you are sensitive and your karma is light, you notice the effects of negativity quickly and easily, the result comes soon. Our karma must be very heavy, because whatever we do, we don't notice it. Therefore, observing karma is very important.

When we talk about taking care of the various vows we have taken—the five precepts, our vows as monks and nuns, our bodhisattva vows—it all has to do with karma. We don't take these ordinations to become prisoners. Therefore, purification is very, very useful.

14

The Qualities of Vajrasattva Are Already Within Us

WHY DOES THE TIBETAN BUDDHIST tradition contain the practice of Vajrasattva?

Everybody would like to be as happy as possible and totally satisfied. We would all like our minds to be clean-clear, controlled, and stable, instead of up and down as they usually are. We would all like to have good concentration, the ability to place our mind on whatever object we choose and have it remain there.

Unfortunately, every day of our lives we are overwhelmed and thrown off balance by the eighty superstitions, or in common Buddhist terms, the three poisonous minds of ignorance, attachment, and hatred. Therefore, we find it hard to be happy. Forget about liberation or enlightenment; we don't even know how to be happy people leading happy lives.

Within us, there is something missing. We are not well balanced; our internal energies are unequal, so our minds are up and down, fluctuating from one extreme to the other. We *are* extreme. We may seem normal from the point of view of the general public, from the New York or Paris point of view, but if you check a little deeper, you will see that we are a little crazy. So, what to do?

We need purification. First, we need to realize, or recognize, our own experiences. Even though they are our own, we are unfamiliar with most of them. To help us understand our own experiences, we need a great deal of purification, and in the Tibetan tradition, the Vajrasattva yoga practice is considered to be one of the most powerful methods of purification.

Who is Heruka Vajrasattva? We consider him to be a manifestation of the unity of fully developed male and female energy, the complete purity of the state of enlightenment. Out of their great compassion and limitless love, the buddhas and bodhisattvas have manifested their collected purity in the archetypal image of Vajrasattva so that we can identify ourselves with him.

We have to understand that the qualities of Vajrasattva are already within us. But our realizations, method, and wisdom are limited. They have to be developed through identification with the limitless, pure energy of the archetype. Instead of thinking of ourselves as limited, hopeless sentient beings, we have to recognize our incredible potential. We can free ourselves from the confusion of uncontrolled concepts. We can develop our consciousness to the limitless states of universal compassion, universal love, universal wisdom, universal freedom. The Vajrasattva practice can lead us beyond ego, beyond grasping, and beyond the dualistic mind. That's what the Vajrasattva practice is about.

Why do we identify with the deity? The deity is the manifestation of the qualities of supreme method and wisdom, so when we unify ourselves with that limitless archetype, we are identifying with those qualities. This leaves no room for our usual limited concepts. Most of you probably know all this, so I don't have to go into detail.

I hope now that you understand why you need to practice the Vajrasattva method. You have to feel that it is very close to you, somehow real, something you can do. That is important. It gives you the courage, space, and freedom you need to cut the limitations that make your life difficult. You know that you can handle, go beyond, be free from those difficulties. That is very important.

Through the experience of purification you can discover that although you might have created a lot of negativity, you are basically a pure person. You might have beaten other sentient beings, your mother, your father; you might hate your friends; you might even want to kill people. We do have negativities. We all live in the sense world. Our egos are in conflict, and we deal with each other with impure energy. The important thing is to overcome all these problems by realizing that since we have made things difficult for ourselves, since we have created our own complications, it is up to us to free ourselves from them. But it is not enough to realize this in a merely intellectual way. We have to gain deep understanding through practice. That way we can really feel that although we have difficulties, we can do something to liberate ourselves from them.

Personally, I feel it is very important that each of us realize and accept that we ourselves are responsible for all negative attitudes and actions.

We, not God or Buddha, created the world's problems. Buddhism does not believe that God created misery. Misery is the creation of the negative, egotistic mind. We have to understand that. If we smash the negative, egotistic mind, we can overcome all problems.

Therefore, we can't blame others for our problems. We created them ourselves. We've created our industrialized society; we've created the Californian life; we've created the New York life; we've created the Paris life. God didn't create them, we did. We've made everything so expensive! A couple of years ago I went shopping in Paris. I couldn't believe how expensive it was. I didn't buy anything. I've been shopping in Ulverston, in Barcelona, where I bought lots of stuff, but I didn't buy anything in Paris. It's all our own doing.

It is very important to recognize how we've created all our own problems. Just understanding this is so important. We've created these problems because we've not been handling our body, speech, and mind correctly. The result has been problems for ourselves, problems for others. We have confused ourselves and others for centuries, millennia, countless lives. It has been this way, it is this way, and it will continue to be this way unless we renounce this cycle of suffering. When you are miserable, you make others miserable. When you are happy, you make others happy.

You have to feel incredulous when you realize the endlessness of all this confusion, and make a strong determination to clear it up: "If I truly love others, if I really have compassion for others, I must improve myself. I must better my behavior, my speech, and my thinking. Without doing so there's no way I can help others. I'm only dreaming if while saying that I want to help others, I merely perpetuate the disastrous actions of my uncontrolled body, speech, and mind."

That's the attitude you need if you want to help others in the best way you can. You're always around other people, aren't you? Even if you go off into the Himalayas, you'll be with people. If you go to where there are no people and try to make friends with the tigers, you'll get eaten up and disappear! So you have to stay around people. We always talk about love. We need love; other sentient beings need love. But our attitudes are childish, and such attitudes make others childish. We need to grow up. Look at what's happening here, even as I speak. With my limited mind, I tell you, "Blah, blah, blah." You take that limited thinking away with you, pass it on to others, and the whole cycle continues to spin. That's the nature of samsara.

However, I am always very happy when people want to practice purification. I truly believe that if religious people really want to practice Dharma, or meditation, the most important thing they can do is to improve their attitude, their actions, and their speech. That is done through the sincere practice of purification.

Most people, especially Westerners, think that they are already pure, that they don't need purification: "I'm pure, I don't have any problems." This is my experience. Many Westerners have come to our Kopan meditation courses, where we teach basic lam-rim, the four noble truths, suffering, and so forth. They tell me straight out, "What are you talking about? You're always going on about problems. I don't have any problems, I'm happy. I've got plenty of money. Why do you keep telling me I'm miserable?" This is the Western mentality. People think that if they've got money, they're happy. From the Buddhist point of view, they're wrong. We think your dollars only make you more miserable.

I'm not saying that only Westerners think like that. Many Asians also think that they're problem-free. But they have problems—they just don't recognize them. They recognize others' problems, but not their own. That's how we are. We see the problems of the people we're with, but we don't see our own. We think we're pure. Such are the limitations of the samsaric mind.

That's why I feel happy when people recognize that they need purification, that there is something they can do to improve their lives. I consider that some kind of realization. You recognize that since your own mind created the negative experiences you have, your own mind can counteract them. This is the main point. Don't think, "I created my own karma. I deserve to suffer in hell." This is completley wrong.

Of course, most of us carry negativities. Our minds are out of control. But we haven't killed people; we haven't killed our parents, or an arhat, or a buddha, so I still think we're lucky. Remember Milarepa. He killed all those people with black magic. Even so, I don't regard him as a criminal, a bad person. On the contrary, I think he's a great person; he set us a good example. He did incredibly negative things, realized black magic was bad, gave it up, practiced pure Dharma, and became completely liberated. Compared to him, we are lucky. We've never killed anybody. But we still have negativities; our minds are still out of control. Yet, we can overcome these problems by practicing the profound methods of tantric yoga.

I feel inspired by Milarepa's attitude. It makes us want to do something, to act. That inspiration itself is liberating. Otherwise we feel, "I'm completely incapable. I'm the most hopeless person in the world. I can't do anything about my motivation or my actions. I'll never be able to change." That's wrong. We can change in any way we like. That's the beauty of the human mind.

Now, before I give this maha-anuttara yoga initiation, I want to remind you that anyone who takes it is making a commitment to retreat on Heruka Vajrasattva for three months. If you have already done this retreat, you don't have to do it again, but if you have retreated on only an aspect of Vajrasattva from one of the lower tantras, you will still have to do the three-month retreat on Heruka Vajrasattva.

However, if you are going back to the West and will have to work, you can do the one hundred thousand mantras as a daily commitment, instead of in retreat, as long as you use the same seat until you've finished, as I have explained elsewhere.[22] I'm sympathetic to that need.

You know, the mantra itself has incredible power. You begin at the level that you're on, but each time you say the mantra, each retreat session, you start to improve. Slowly, slowly, the mantra elevates you. Even though you might not have deep concentration, just trying to visualize and repeating the mantra has what I would dare to call a miraculous effect on you. Without your even trying, the mantra touches your deep subconscious and purifies you. There is nothing at all worldly, contaminated, or evil about the mantra; it has an inherent power to elevate that automatically burns up your impure, garbage energy. That's the great beauty of mantra. You don't have to be a great meditator to benefit from it. Mantra can automatically elevate you from your ordinary way of thinking and speak to you in a place beyond heavy worldly concepts. That gives you the space to see things more clearly, and that is good enough.

Mantra is also a kind of secret language. Normally, we communicate on a very low level. When we argue with each other, we're on a low energy plane. Our quarrels are very worldly. Mantra takes you away from the things that usually drive you crazy, from the things in which you are normally involved. It sort of hypnotizes you into communicating with higher levels of mind by blocking normal, conventional, low level communication. That's another way in which mantra is very helpful. Of course, mere words can never explain the true nature of mantra.

Another thing: we don't consider Vajrasattva and the mantra to be two separate things. The Vajrasattva mantra *is* Vajrasattva; Vajrasattva *is* the Vajrasattva mantra. Buddhism is set up for us to transform our ordinary body, speech, and mind into those of an enlightened being. By emanating as the deity, we transform our body; by reciting the mantra, we transform our speech; and by generating bodhicitta and the wisdom of sunyata, we transform our mind.

Vajrasattva is not simply for purification. The visualization you do is a process to help you generate wisdom and compassion and to experience something akin to what you would experience in completion stage practice. You visualize Vajrasattva above the crown of your head in union with his consort. From their heart chakras, blissful white kundalini energy rushes all the way down their shushumas and comes out where they are joined at their secret chakras. It continues down through the lotus and moon seat, through your crown chakra and down your shushuma, and you practice the various purifying meditation techniques. You then unify and identify with Vajrasattva. You experience enlightened energy. This is not just a purification practice.

Some people think visualization is a bit funny; that when you visualize you are just making something up. I think it is a most powerful method; a powerful method to break your ordinary concepts, your preconceptions. I cannot just tell you, "You are wrong, you are wrong. Your way of thinking is wrong; you are so deluded." Those are just words. You have to experience for yourself, "How deluded I am, how I project things." You have to see for yourself how different projections make you feel and affect your view of reality. Vajrasattva introduces you to the way you think, the way you interpret the reality of yourself and your world. That's what visualization shows you. The visualization of Vajrasattva is a teaching on sunyata.

I can listen to teachings on sunyata twenty-four hours a day, seven days a week, for a year, "Sunyata, sunyata, sunyata, ego is bad, wrong view…," listening, listening, somebody is up there teaching me. But in the end, I'll still be full of concepts and thoughts. In just the shortest time, Vajrasattva visualization can completely shut down your mental chatter, giving you the space to work out what you see. I really believe that this is a much stronger way to introduce you to sunyata, with your own experience, your own language, your own mind, and your own thinking. I'm probably wrong, but that's what I believe. Really, this is most powerful.

Basically, I'm a skeptic. I don't believe things easily. I didn't expect that Vajrasattva meditation would do much for the Western mind. I just observed what was happening. So far, I think that Vajrasattva retreat has been an unprecedented success among my Western students. Their minds have definitely changed for the better. Without retreat, their minds would not have changed. It takes a strong retreat to change Westerners' minds. Then something really happens. The evidence of this experience has convinced me that the Vajrasattva practice really works for Westerners.

15

Action Is Everything

We have to act, not just philosophize. Philosophical concepts may be able to correct wrong ideas, erroneous ways of thought, and mistaken beliefs, but intellectual correction is not enough. Along with that we need a powerful force to channel our minds into the correct, divine philosophy of the middle way.

For example, Lord Buddha taught that we should avoid extremes and follow the middle way, because going to extremes and avoiding everything would make us sick. He said that we should adjust our lives both relatively and absolutely. But these statements are still views, ideas, and opinions, aren't they? Our lives should be more active than that. When you get your hands dirty, touch the earth, plant seeds, and water the ground, green plants manifest organically. Vajrasattva practice is a lot like that.

The Vajrasattva meditation is not complicated; it's very simple and easy to understand. It's not something that takes a lot of intellectual thought. You just do it, just act. That is what we need. Transformation never comes without action. No matter how much you study and learn, how much information you collect, it is action that really helps you integrate your life. The Tibetan Buddhist tradition contains a wide range of preliminary practices (*ngön-dro*). Vajrasattva is one of these. Even though it is very simple and practical, it is one of the most powerful methods of purification we have.

At first I was very skeptical that a method that worked for Easterners would also work for Westerners, but I have now seen hundreds of Westerners retreat on Vajrasattva with great success and great improvement in their minds. This experience has both amazed and satisfied me, and there is no doubt that it is highly worthwhile.

Buddhism always emphasizes meditation, mindfulness, awareness, method, and wisdom. Every word of the teachings points you in the direction of insight. The Vajrasattva yoga method is a very simple means of showing you who you are. It reveals your shortcomings and your strengths and is especially helpful in ripping off the heavy blanket of wrong conceptions that prevents you from seeing the reality of yourself. Even if you find it difficult to meditate or have poor concentration, this practice can give you inner satisfaction and a real taste of Buddhadharma. Therefore, it is very useful.

Normally, our motivation is at a very low level, and our actions are quite mundane. Sometimes I feel as though we're dealing with the hell realm in our human relationships. Well, that may be a bit of an exaggeration, but what I mean is that we don't use our human intelligence enough. Vajrasattva meditation brings you up from those lower levels of mind to a higher, more human plane of consciousness. You just have to do it, that's all.

Furthermore, the practice is structured so that while you are working with and meditating on the sadhana at a conscious level, positive energy from your subconscious mind is being activated and drawn upon to enhance your practice. This is one of the psychological features of tantra and one of the reasons that it is so powerful. Tantra liberates you by working at both the conscious and subconscious levels to lead your mind into the gradual path to enlightenment.

Most of us are limited when it comes to recognizing both the male and female aspects of our being. Vajrasattva meditation demonstrates the magnificent blissful unified energy within us. We need this. We feel lonely because we are unaware of the totality of the inner human environment. And as long as we follow our monkey minds, we'll remain unaware of it and continue to feel lonely. Vajrasattva shows you what it's like to be a complete person, an emanation of totality. This is very helpful.

The Vajrasattva mantra is especially powerful. I call it "miraculous television"! On regular television you see incredible things, don't you? All sorts of samsaric things can manifest on your screen. Similarly, mantra is like divine television. By simply reciting the mantra, you bring the three principal aspects of the path—renunciation, bodhicitta, and right view—come into your stream of consciousness. Divine pride and clarity also enter. Mantra is very powerful because it gives you access to levels of consciousness that are far beyond the ordinary, mundane, lower levels on which you usually operate.

Intellectually oriented people find it difficult to transform themselves because they think that the way to perfection is through their intellect: "This is knowledge; this is the liberator; intellect is everything." Intellect is not everything—action is everything. For example, if a simple person who doesn't have great intellectual learning gets into a jet plane, he still gets to wherever he wants to go. Similarly, if someone who has not studied Dharma extensively climbs aboard the jet of the Vajrasattva yoga method, he or she can be carried to transformation without having to worry about accumulating intellectual knowledge.

Our problem is that we are too intellectual. We say, "This is no good; I don't want that; I want the other." That's how we choose, and that's our problem. Our intellect causes most of our dissatisfaction. We have taken so many intellectual trips in our life, yet we are still dissatisfied. You can see this most clearly in the West.

The nuclear essence of tantra is that the human being is the deity. The human being *is* the god; the human being *is* the deity. I have to emphasize this. We have the qualities of the deity within us. You always think that the deity is something rarefied and inaccessible, but through tantra you can touch the deity, recognize yourself as the deity. That's why it is very powerful.

Buddhism teaches that the basic human problem is the ridiculous thought that we are hopeless. This way of identifying ourselves damages our human quality. Therefore, we need to discover the divinity within us, the divine qualities that are already there. Buddhism is really so realistic, so scientific, so down-to-earth, so clean-clear: human beings *do* have a pure nature and divine inner qualities, so they should recognize and unify with them. And according to Lord Buddha, the way to recognize our divine qualities is not simply to *know* that they are there, but to act, to act. The way to act is to practice tantra. Tantra is not about words; the essence of tantra is action.

Of course, I'm not a great meditator; nor have I had much experience. I'm somewhat narrow and out of touch with reality. Nevertheless, I have done mantra retreats and, miraculously, have experienced to a certain extent things that I have never experienced when not in retreat. I have discovered new dimensions to life, a new reality. Mantra has the power to take you into a new dimension, a new space. That is what tantra and mantra can do.

Sometimes these new experiences can shock you because they are so different from your normal reality. On the other hand, you can experience clean-clear visions that are very real for you. Anyway, I'm not going to try to explain all this. I just want to say that is is extremely worthwhile for you to act. Action is simple and direct. I'm telling you all this because many would-be practitioners get confused by the many teachings and practices they find in Buddhism. They don't know what to do, what practices are for them. Consequently, they don't do anything properly. If you can concentrate on certain meditation practices and be very focused when you do them, I can guarantee that you will change for the better.

Therefore, when I give the Vajrasattva initiation, I don't make you commit to doing the practice or reciting the mantra every day of your life, but I do ask most of you to do a three-month group retreat. The only purpose of making a retreat commitment is to ensure that you have some experience, that you are not just spiritually grasping but are doing something to elevate yourself. People who have already done the retreat have already gained the experience and don't necessarily have to do it again.

I understand that life in the West does not always allow you to go off for a three-month retreat, so I sometimes make an exception. If you don't have time to do the strict retreat, you can practice at home for an hour a day until you have recited the required number of mantras. You should try to finish within two to three years.

The main condition here is that you sit in the same seat. Usually our minds are fickle; we can't focus intensively and are completely distracted, constantly looking for something new, something different. This is an unhealthy attitude. You lose penetrative insight; you lose intensive awareness. It's not that a constantly changing environment drives you crazy, but it does spoil your meditation. A stable situation promotes simplicity, clarity, insight, and intensive awareness. If we were beyond conditioning, it would be all right, but our minds are at a lower level, where conditions affect us. Everything affects us: stars, poisonous plants, snakes, human beings, colors. Consciously or unconsciously, we are affected. To overcome this tendency, we meditate in the same place.

However, I think I have to make another compromise here to accommodate a lifestyle such as that in America, where people move around a lot. Make a small meditation box that will fit into your car. Then when you move house, you can take your seat with you. The continuity of daily practice is very important, so please don't break it—wherever you go, take your meditation box with you.

Continuity is really important. We have all had moments of sensitive, intensive awareness where we could almost hear the flowers breathe; perfect, blissful, satisfied experiences where we have never wanted to look at anything else. But what we have lacked is that state of total satisfaction; our intensive awareness has been interrupted. We are always on, off, on, off, up, down, and that's the problem. In fact, the Tibetan word for tantra, *gyüd,* means continuity, and continuity is very important if you want to stay happy. If you reach a certain state of happiness and satisfaction, you want to maintain it, don't you? You don't want to fill your consciousness with disasters. This is so simple, so logical. We *can* be logical at times. The problem is that when we are off, we are illogical, and it is only when we are on that logic prevails. It is important to maintain the continuity of happy conditions without allowing misery to interrupt. Continuous practice is therefore very important.

Retreat is very special. The literal meaning of the Tibetan word for retreat, *tsam,* is isolation. But isolation from what—reality? Well, we're already isolated from that. We need to isolate ourselves from mentally or externally confused situations, any circumstances that tend to make us unclear. If you can avoid all that for the duration of your retreat, transformation will come of itself, without your even having to worry about it. And as I said before, if you can't isolate yourself in strict retreat, the continuity of daily practice is very important. If one day you are busy and can't manage your usual session, do half an hour. If that's too much, do twenty minutes, or ten, or even five. There has to some continuity. Your stream of consciousness is like a highway, so keep the energy flowing along it.

Buddha manifests in the radiant white form of Vajrasattva. Why does Buddha manifest in different ways? Because different sentient beings have different needs, and Buddha himself said that he would manifest in various forms in accordance with those needs. We believe that he can appear as Krishna, as Jesus, as a woman, as tea, as a criminal—in whatever form will benefit each sentient being, to fulfill whatever needs we have.

In order to dispel the darkness of ignorance, Lord Buddha manifests the totality of his pure energy in a radiant white body. You can see for yourself that when you are confused and negative, your mind gets very dark. The blissful radiant white emanation of Vajrasattva purifies that darkness.

When you practice the Vajrasattva meditation you should not feel discouraged, "Oh, I can't do it perfectly." What is perfect? You have to build up to perfection from the level you're on. You build your dream home on an empty piece of land; here you build up perfect energy from the emptiness of sunyata. Just do your best according to your own ability and don't expect too much. Lord Buddha doesn't expect everyone to be at the same level. We might all be doing Vajrasattva meditation, using the same words, the same method, but each of us has his own understanding, her own conscious realm. Buddhism understands that. So don't worry about trying to be the same as your neighbor. Just take it easy, keep yourself clean-clear, and do what you can. That's good enough.

When you take the Vajrasattva initiation you should have a strong motivation and no doubts. Motivation is the nuclear essence of liberation. The right attitude will set you free. When you take the initiation, you should not be seeking the short-term pleasures of beach and ice-cream. You should instead have the strong intention to make your life as beneficial as possible for others. This is the most important factor in taking the Vajrasattva initiation. And I think that you already have that motivation. Don't think, "Oh, that doesn't sound like me." You can definitely purify all negativities of your ordinary body, speech, and mind and thereby discover the vajra body, speech, and mind.

[Lama Yeshe gives the initiation.]

Now the initiation has nearly finished. According to Tibetan tradition, at this point the lama touches each disciple's crown with the torma that represents the deity, as I have explained on an earlier occasion. I think this may have been a Tibetan innovation and not something that came down from ancient times. Lamas are very kind and not so busy, so they try to put all their energy into the Dharma path. They make tormas, transform them into the deity through meditation, and then place them on the disciples' heads to ensure they experience Vajrasattva descending to their hearts. I'm not going to do this today. I've got nothing against the practice, but we're in the West, and I think Vajrasattva is already in your heart, so it's not necessary.

You can see that the Vajrasattva practice is very simple, but if you find it difficult to visualize the deity above the crown of your head, you can visualize Vajrasattva at your brow chakra. If this is still too hard, instead of visualizing him in the usual form of the deity, you can visualize at your brow chakra a white OM on a moon disc surrounded by the mantra standing counterclockwise around its edge. As you concentrate on the OM and the mantra, blissful energy emantes from them and fills your entire nervous system, forcing out all the garbage of your impurities, especially those of your body.

You should be able to feel your impurities. If you can't, it may well mean that you have already achieved a certain degree of purity. "Pure" and "impure" are not simply dependent upon your belief, not necessarily just religious ideas. In your mind there is a kind of substantial psychological entity that depends upon your conventional mode of thought. This is what determines purity and impurity, and you should be able to detect it.

Similarly, at your throat chakra there is a red AH on a moon disc, surrounded by the mantra, and at your heart, a blue HUM on a moon disc, surrounded by the mantra. When you recite the mantra, blissful energy emanates as before and purifies your negativities of speech and mind, respectively. So, instead of just sitting there feeling lonely, miserable, and incapable of doing the meditation with the complete visualization, you can practice this simplified form. It works; it really opens you up.

The main commentary will tell you most of what you need to know to do the Vajrasattva retreat. If you study it, you will see how worthwhile and effective for your mind retreat really can be. Retreat is not a joke. All of us need to make the time and space to elevate our minds. If we don't do this for ourselves, how will we ever develop our human potential? Also, students who have completed the retreat can help explain the commentary to you.

After your retreat it is good for you to do the Dorje Khadro fire puja, although this is not a commitment. Some people feel upset that they did not do the retreat as well as they might have, that they didn't recite the mantra properly, or something like that. The fire puja burns all those doubts away, leaving you clean-clear and satisfied with what you did.

Let me emphasize again the benefit of short sessions. Do your practice intensively and well and you'll enjoy it; you'll leave your meditation seat wanting to come back. It somehow retains the energy of your positive mental vibrations. This helps to make your retreat easy.

I think it is wonderful that you people want to practice purification. There is so much impure energy around the planet these days, so much contamination of various sorts. It is rare that anyone even knows about purification, let alone thinks about practicing it. You are so brave. I am very pleased that you to want to purify your miserable energy and have a happy life. Also, purifying yourselves properly benefits mankind. That's all we can do. I feel blissful that you are serious in wanting to purify yourself, that you are not hypocritical, and that we are not wasting our time. I would even go so far as to say that even if you are not going to act, just wanting to purify yourself is enough for me. You touch my heart. Thank you so much!

Part 4

Heruka Vajrasattva Tsok

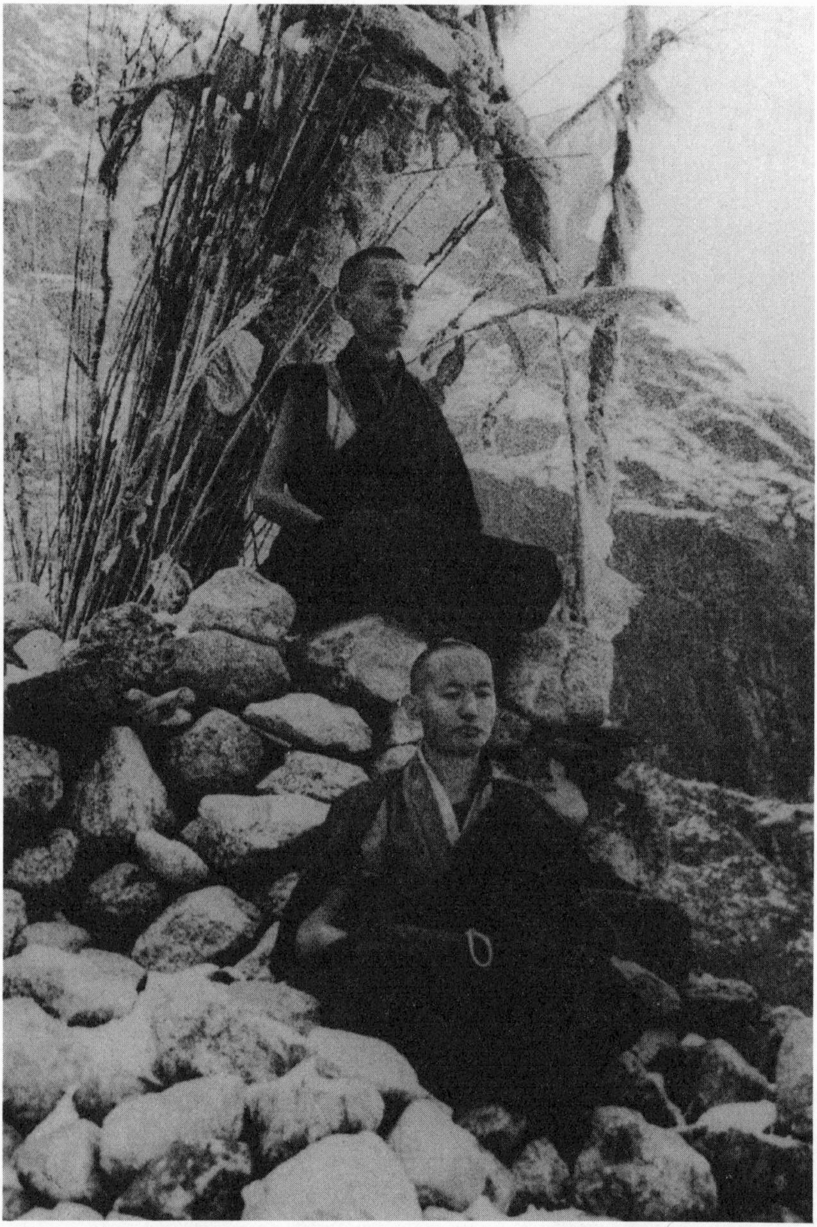

Photographer unknown

16

WHAT IS TSOK?

TSOK MEANS GATHERING. We gather together the things that we're offering, and we ourselves gather together to do the practice. Gathering together with other practitioners, concentrating our minds into the same space, gives us great inspiration. It's much better than just doing a puja alone in our own rooms. This is the Tibetan connotation of tsok.

An example from my college at Sera likens group puja to a straw broom. You can't sweep much floor with just one straw, but when many straws are gathered together to make a broom, you can clean an entire assembly hall in no time at all. We are not as strong as distinguished practitioners such as Milarepa. He was okay all by himself; we're not ready for that yet.

So it's good that we come together trying to develop single-pointedness of mind; one hundred people's minds all meeting at the same place. This becomes very powerful.

Tsok in the Tibetan tradition is a most profound method of purification, a profound way of gaining realizations. When you recite the text in English you can see how many subjects are included in the practice. The *Guru Puja*, for example, covers the entire path to enlightenment from beginning to end. So it can happen that in your daily meditations on the lam-rim you're not making any obvious progress, when suddenly during a puja, because of the conducive atmosphere you've created, zoom!—some realization comes into your mind. Many people have gained realizations during puja simply because of the atmosphere.

Normally, we push ourselves to achieve, but nothing happens because we've not made the space for something to happen. By gathering together to offer tsok we're making space. When the right space opens, zoom!—realizations come as if magnetically attracted. This is true.

Therefore, it's important to put yourself into the right atmosphere when you're practicing a sadhana or anything else. You might have done a particular puja one hundred times before, but somehow you have never reached quite the right spot. When, at a certain point, you do reach the right spot, zoom!—something happens. To grow, we need the right atmosphere.

In the philosophical terminology of Buddhism, we talk about karma: "Create good karma, and you'll get this or that good result." I'm simply going to say that to get the results you want, you have to create the right atmosphere. If you build a greenhouse, flowers will grow and they'll also be protected from damage by hail. It's the same thing with our baby minds. We need to create the proper environment in which they can develop, and we also need to protect them. Our gathering together for puja, giving each other energy, is the kind of protection our minds require.

In the Tibetan tradition of Mahayana Buddhism we're always talking about the benefits we derive from all mother sentient beings. Take this Darjeeling tea we drink. Think how many people were involved in its getting here: the growers, the pickers, the sorters, the packagers, the shippers, the shopkeepers, our own cooks...finally, we get to drink it here. You know from your lam-rim studies that, directly or indirectly, every sentient being has helped you get that cup of tea. And not just that cup of tea. All our happiness, from the lowest samsaric pleasure to the eternal bliss of liberation and enlightenment, comes from each of us to the other.

Thus, to gain realizations we need to create the right atmosphere. We do this by gathering together and directing our minds to the same place. The power of this practice brings understanding. I think it's great: we're an international gathering, and each of us has developed in our own unique way; but despite our differences, our minds can still meet at the same place, and we can communicate with each other. I really think it's wonderful. Parents may not be able to communicate with their children, but here we are, from different countries all over the world, and we're able to communicate with each other, heart to heart.

Another connotation of tsok is "party"—a party at which we share simultaneously born great wisdom and bliss. Now *that's* a party!

17

Heruka Vajrasattva Tsok: The First Commentary

When I was selecting a title for this tsok offering, I had many names to choose from, but somehow I thought "An Antidote to the Vajra Hells" was the most suitable. Many of my students have done the Heruka Vajrasattva retreat, which is an extremely powerful way of purifying all one's negative energy. Therefore, when I was asked if we could offer tsok under the bodhi tree here in Bodhgaya,[23] I thought it appropriate to write a short tsok offering to Heruka Vajrasattva.

We call this offering a banquet because it is like a great blissful party to which we invite from the ten directions the buddhas, bodhisattvas, dakas, dakinis, and whatever other pure manifestations we would like to be there.

The offering ingredients

Any kind of food and drink can be offered as tsok. You don't have to offer Tibetan-style tormas made of tsampa—they didn't do that in ancient India back in Nagarjuna's time. You can offer carrots, chocolate, milk shakes, or even black foods, such as onions, garlic, and radish—anything you like; whatever is clean and available where you live. If you are an exceptionally strong tantric practitioner you can even offer unclean things, such as excrement, but since we are not that advanced, it is better for us to make clean offerings.

The merit field

First verse. Since this is a tantric practice, before we actually offer the tsok, we first have to transform our ordinary view of the environment and all the beings in it. Visualize yourself, the other people offering the tsok together with you, the offering ingredients—in fact, everything—as manifestations of the totally unified great bliss and wisdom of non-duality. Then, in the space in front of you, from non-dual bliss and emptiness, the Vajrasattva mandala appears, with Heruka Vajrasattva and his consort at its center.

Following its natural tendency, our narrow mind will visualize this mandala as small and crowded, but it is not. The mandala occupies all of space and is filled with infinite objects of offering, which are in the nature of blissful nectar and transcendental wisdom. You should transform your offering—whether it be just one orange or a table full of food—into infinite offerings filling space: billions of oranges, apple,s and so forth. Sometimes I visualize and offer a cosmic Western supermarket—a much better offering than some limited, third-world vegetable market! Your offering should be limitless. Even if you are offering only one object, infinite objects of the five senses, all in the nature of bliss, emanate from it.

Second verse. The usual perception we have of ourselves and others is very ordinary. When, for example, we gather to offer tsok, we see ourselves as hopeless, pathetic individuals surrounded by other hopeless, pathetic individuals, all striving earnestly to make some kind of offering. From the tantric point of view, offerings made like that don't work. That is not the way to offer tsok. You should feel that all those around you are your dear friends—even those with whom you might be fighting at present—and see each of them as a Vajrasattva of radiant white light. You can do it. One of the great beauties of being human is that you can change your mind at any time. It is flexible, and you can develop the skill of changing bad situations into good.

Thus, in the sphere of great non-dual bliss all beings appear as male and female deities—dakas and dakinis. Their appearance is like an illusion, as if it had been created by a magician. Have you ever had the experience of being somewhere, watching many different people of various nationalities, shapes, and sizes passing by, and feeling as if it were a dream or an illusion? When offering this tsok, you should transform all beings into the aspect of Vajrasattva and regard your entire visualization as illusory. Actually, the way we see each other is already illusory, even though we think we are all so solid and so real.

Some of the dakas and dakinis we visualize are extremely peaceful and blissful in appearance; others are in the aspect of granting development; some manifest power; others, great wrath. They all seem to be dancing.

You should consider that you yourselves dance whenever you go anywhere. In a way, whenever you go to the movies, to a restaurant, back home, you *are* dancing. When offering tsok, you should visualize the dakas and dakinis as very active and alive—really doing things to benefit all mother sentient beings—not dull, inactive, and dead. They manifest in all these different ways for the benefit of all sentient beings, embodying not partial and disjointed, but fully developed and totally unified, method and wisdom.

All tsok gatherings, for example, the *Guru Puja*, are based on transformation. First you generate non-dual transcendental great bliss and wisdom, and then everything—all actions, the offering ingredients, yourselves, the guru to whom you are making the offering—arises from that. At these times you should not see any living beings as suffering sick people, cripples, hungry ghosts, and so forth. Everything that appears should look transcendental and evoke great bliss. Therefore, it is best that here you visualize all beings as Vajrasattvas. It is really excellent if, during the one hour or whatever time it takes you to make the tsok offering, you can control your mind and prevent garbage-like ordinary concepts from arising. Usually such thoughts fully occupy our minds, causing us much confusion and making us more deluded than ever. How wonderful it would be if for just one hour your mind could give no space for self-pity to arise.

BLESSING THE INNER OFFERINGS

(OM KHANDA ROHI...) Here we bless the offering ingredients. The deity Khandarohi has one face and four arms and, if possible, should be visualized dispelling interfering spirits and so forth. It does not matter if you cannot make this visualization, but you should at least sprinkle some inner offering nectar on the offering ingredients and feel that all negative, miserly spirits have been driven away. "Spirits" does not refer only to outer hindrances but also to any negative energy within you that pollutes your offering. This energy, too, is purified.

(OM SVABHAVA...) We call this the sunyata mantra. Recognizing the sunyata, or emptiness of inherent existence, of the offering ingredients is a very powerful way of purifying ordinary conceptions and negative energy. It is essential to do this in order to make a proper tsok offering.

The seed syllable OM symbolizes the divine vajra body, which is union-oneness with the divine vajra speech and mind. SVABHAVA means natural, not artificial; SHUDDHA (and SHUDDHO) mean pure; SARVA means all; DHARMA means existent phenomena; and HAM means I am, which is to be felt with divine pride. These Sanskrit words contain a profound explanation of the pure, fundamental nature of human beings and all other phenomena. The mantra means: all existent phenomena are inherently pure [not in the relative but in the absolute sense] and so am I.

You have to understand your real nature. Most of the time you are unnatural. With intelligence your ego produces anger and desire; this is the wrong sort of intelligence. Your ego creates an artificial image of yourself, and you believe, "This is me; how beautiful (or ugly) I am." Then you present this false image of yourself to others. As long as you are under the control of your ego you are not natural. Therefore, you have to listen to and touch your fundamental, true nature. If you can do this, you will touch purity. Thus, the usual human self-pitying wrong conception—"I am hopeless; I am impure; I am bad; I cannot do anything; I cannot help myself"—is completely false and the exact opposite of what the sunyata mantra is saying.

Your nature is not what your negative projections believe. Buddha explains that it is mistaken to think that you are really evil or sinful. Your fundamental nature is pure. The artificial cloud that your ego produces is not your true nature but a fabrication dreamed up by your ego. Therefore, be natural.

It is very easy to see how we are not natural. Look at how people's behavior changes with their ideas. Take, as a simple example, the way people walk. As their self-image changes, so does the way they walk. You can see this for yourself. Young people project a certain image of themselves, believe they have to act accordingly, and walk and dress the way they think they should. Old people do not understand why the young are acting like that, criticize them, and the generation gap widens.

All this is completely artificial. Act naturally. The sunyata mantra shows that the true nature of human beings is positive. You should not believe in your ego-projected negative self-image. Buddha explained clearly how all your suffering comes from your ego, and that's why Buddhism always teaches how destructive the ego's projections are.

In sunyata meditation you listen to your inner self, go beyond artificial thoughts, become tranquil and peaceful, and touch the fundamental reality of your being. Thus, sunyata meditation cuts all the concepts that make you miserable, especially the idea that you are somehow permanent and inherently self-existent. If these wrong beliefs are not cut off but merely suppressed, the symptoms they produce will keep on recurring. You might be able to control one kind of suffering, but another will arise in its stead.

Whether or not you recite the sunyata mantra, it is imperative that you see that the self-image held by your self-pity does not exist. I could explain this in deep philosophical terms, but I prefer to keep it simple. Think back a year to the "I am this" you were holding at that time and compare it with the "I am this" you hold today. Has the "I" that you feel changed at all or not? Careful analysis will reveal that although some things have changed, the I that you feel today is identical with the I you felt a year ago. You can see how wrong, both relatively and absolutely, this feeling is.

All phenomena are changing from moment to moment—there is no way for our I to remain unchanged. When you realize how your ego-grasping ignorance has been clinging to its nonsensical self-identity, believing, for example, that the you of ten years ago is still here today, you will laugh at how deluded you have been. Buddha always taught that we are deluded. Being deluded means holding nonsensical, hallucinatory conceptions. Even if you have been meditating for twenty or thirty years, if your meditation has not begun to shake your ego and destroy these ideas, you have not been meditating properly. The more extreme your ego's self-identity, the more solid your ego appears, and the tighter you hang on to it. When you shake your ego to its roots you create an earthquake that causes the Mount Meru of your samsaric mandala to crumble.

Buddha's teaching on universal reality is profound. It shows humans the best way to be healthy. It breaks all concepts, shatters all illusions. Buddha even said that if you hold to a fixed conception of *him,* you are trapped. Spiritual seekers of today, under the control of their egos, grasp at their self-existent gurus, saying, "I love you; you are a wonderful guru. Do you love me? You should." Buddha would have rejected disciples who thought like that. He did not want anybody to grasp at either himself or his teachings. If you are attached to even the paramita path or tantra, you are trapped, you are foolish. You cannot be healthy. There are no exceptions in terms of what you should not grasp at. You should not grasp at samsaric phenomena; you should not grasp at Dharma. That is Lord Buddha's prescription for perfect health.

These days many gurus seem to be attached to their disciples and want their disciples to be attached to them. This is completely wrong. It is most unhealthy for disciples to be attached to either their teacher or their path. Buddha wants you to be healthy, happy forever, and free from all concepts and doctrines, from all bondage. Therefore, you have to recognize as false all concepts of the "you" of the past that you are holding right now, and break them down. In the gloom of this ignorance you are deceived by the seductive dance of the objects of the five senses. But when you recognize the way your ego cheats you, it will no longer be able to do so. If you really understand this, you will understand sunyata.

The profound sunyata mantra tells you that the true nature of yourself and all other phenomena is one. But your ego divides, separates, and categorizes everything so that you can never really be close to anything. Even after a lifetime together, husbands and wives are not really close and do not understand each other because their egos have kept them apart.

The mantra states that in reality all existent phenomena are one and "HAM," "so am I." Ultimately you are pure, one with all existence; therefore, generate divine pride. When you experience sunyata, you become one with all phenomena, inseparable, like milk poured into milk. When you realize sunyata, your dualistic mind vanishes. It is dualistic because it divides everything into two—for example, "me" and "you." When you realize your own ultimate nature and mine, there will be no distinction between us.

People in the world protest so much about racism and stage political demonstrations against it, sometimes getting killed in the process. From the Buddhist point of view, racism will continue to exist as long as the dualistic mind has not been eradicated. Until you have discovered ultimate reality, the unity of all existence, all talk of abolishing racism is just a joke. Buddha gave the perfect, practical method of integration, which we all can experience in our daily lives. The great beauty of being human is that we can transcend the relative world and experience the absolute.

All becomes empty... The skull cup we visualize here is not one of the small ones we use in pujas. It should be huge; the bigger the better. It contains the five meats and the five nectars. You are in the aspect of Vajrasattva. From the HUM at your heart, a beam of light shines into the skullcup, heating its contents and melting them into a vast ocean of inexhaustible blissful nectar.

Whenever you offer tsok, you have to recognize the blissful nature of whatever you offer. For example, oranges might appear as oranges, but in essence they are blissful nectar. And the deity to whom you are offering the tsok—in this case Vajrasattva—does not just munch it up like we do but, instead, extracts the essence of the tsok, great bliss, through a thin straw of light that he sends out from his tongue. You too should recognize all the offerings, and indeed all your everyday food and drink, as being in the nature of great bliss.

Then, saying the mantra OM AH HUM HA HO HRI three times, you bless the tsok.

This pure offering... Reciting this verse helps your mind avoid energizing superstition.

VERSE ONE

Here we offer the tsok with a request to develop within us the simultaneously born great bliss and wisdom, the unique tantric path to enlightenment.

Recite the Heruka Vajrasattva mantra once after each verse. If you recite it clearly, evenly, and at the right speed you will purify millions of lives' negativity. Sometimes you feel so heavy with non-virtue that you almost cannot move; you feel as if you are drowning in a vast ocean of negativity. And once you have decided that you feel heavy, you feel heavy! Buddhist psychology makes the point that if you believe that you are negative, you become negative. If I project that you are hopeless, to me you manifest as hopeless. We should not think like that. We have powerful methods of purifying even the most serious downfalls—for example, broken root vows of tantra. It is the experience of many great yogis that the Vajrasattva practice can purify all negative energy. There is no negativity that Vajrasattva meditation cannot purify. It is very important for you to understand this. You already have a very low opinion of yourself. You should not make it worse when you encounter religion. This is wrong. Of course, you should recognize your shortcomings, but at the same time you should give yourself inspiration by always remembering your potential to become a buddha.

VERSE TWO

How do we make our precious human rebirth useless? By clinging to the pleasures of the objects of the five senses. Why? Because our sense consciousnesses are hallucinating. We have to purify their impure, dualistic vision. We are too concerned about the welfare of just this life. For example, look at what happens when you go to India for a Dharma festival. You are full of good intentions, but when you arrive, you get upset because there's no good food, tea, or coffee. Of course, you have to make sure your body remains healthy, but even when it is, the lack of amenities disturbs you. You say you want liberation, enlightenment, and to help others, but in reality, your mind is completely obsessed with your own pathetic, ego-determined pleasures. Such exaggerated concern for the happiness of this life alone must be eliminated; it only makes you progressively narrower. It is completely untrue that this life's happiness is all there is to strive for.

Students put a great deal of effort into studying hard so that they will pass their examinations and get a job. They may enjoy certain diversionary pleasures while doing so, but these are secondary to their main purpose. They do not allow the small pleasures to prevent them from attaining their main goal. In the same way, you who seek the highest goal of everlasting satisfaction should be strongly dedicated to that and prepared to sacrifice the comfort of this life for it. Without sacrificing attachment to samsaric pleasures you cannot gain liberation. Also, when you make a definite decision to strive for liberation knowing that there will be sacrifices to make, you will experience a kind of bliss whenever you encounter obstacles. All ego conflicts and suffering come from the poison of clinging to the ordinary concepts and appearances of this life. When we offer the tsok with this verse, we request blessings to enable us to abandon such clinging.

VERSE THREE

This verse shows how you create bad karma and add to your delusions. Improper attention, whose nature is superstition, produces more superstition. Acting under its influence you create bad karma. All these things are like a heavy blanket covering your mind and, along with the demon of the impure, dualistic view, have to be purified.

Here we request blessings to develop perfect renunciation of samsara in our hearts. To achieve true renunciation it is not enough just to have strong aversion to samsara. You have to investigate how improper attention generates superstition, thus fueling samsara. The dualistic improper attention has to be purified. Then you can develop renunciation.

Some monks and nuns seem to think that they became arhats the moment they were ordained. You can't become an arhat in a day. Some lay people also seem to think that monks and nuns should be arhats, and criticize them as soon as they do something wrong: "Oh, look at those monks; they're no better than me." It is easy to criticize the Sangha. You can even criticize the Buddha: "He was so selfish, going off alone to meditate for six years." I do not believe that the renunciation of monks and nuns is necessarily any better than that of lay people. But at least monks and nuns have recognized what they need to do to overcome their samsaric difficulties and are trying to develop renunciation. That is the right thing to do. They may not be arhats, but they are doing the best they can.

As you know from studying the middle level teachings on the graduated path to enlightenment, where it explains the causes of samsara and how to get rid of them, it is difficult to achieve perfect renunciation. We have difficulty renouncing samsara because our superstitions cause us to create more and more karma, and as a result, our blanket of obscurations gets thicker and thicker. Therefore, we pray to Guru Vajrasattva to help us purify all this.

VERSE FOUR

You also know from the sutra teachings how the dualistic mind of self-cherishing is the foundation of all suffering and the principal evil. We make this offering to purify self-cherishing and to generate the most perfect bodhicitta in our hearts.

VERSE FIVE

All phenomena are labeled—given names—by superstition; as a result, they exist. But our superstitious minds are not content to leave it at that. For example, when you see a beautiful object, which exists as a beautiful object merely as a projection of your superstitious mind, you do not just let it be, but try to make its beauty concrete, self-existent, special. This is again the dualistic vision and has to be purified. Thus, we make this offering with the request that we might realize the mahamudra, the great seal of emptiness.

VERSE SIX

In life, as soon as I consider other people to be ordinary and bothersome, my problems start. I begin to disrespect them and put them down. All this arises from ordinary concepts, my superstitious mind. According to tantric philosophy, there are eighty superstitions, some of which are gross and others, subtle. All of them have to be purified. We also have to purify the impure dualistic vision, which is likened to a strong hurricane that causes planes to crash and destroys houses and property. Thus, we offer the nectar tsok, whose nature is that of the wisdom of the five dhyani buddhas, to Guru Vajrasattva, requesting the blessings of the four actual initiations.

Why are we asking for more initiations when we have already received so many? Actually, the question is: have we really received *any* initiations? It is very difficult to receive a real initiation. It is not something that you simply get from a lama. In my opinion—and I hope this does not sound too extreme—in an initiation, the disciple is more important than the guru.

Although I say it is very difficult to receive the four actual initiations, I do not mean that you have necessarily received nothing. The initiation you receive is determined by your level of understanding. In a gathering of two hundred people, no two have the same experience. And although the lama gives all four initiations, probably nobody receives them all. Some people might feel that they have received nothing and will ask their friends, "Did I receive the initiation?" This is something you have to judge for yourself; nobody else can tell you what you have received. However, it is extremely rare for someone to really receive the four initiations.

Also, the degree to which you receive an initiation depends upon the deity concerned and the conditions under which the ceremony is performed. You have a strong karmic connection with some deities and a weaker one with others. And I say that the conditions affect your experience because I am talking about the relative initiation, not the absolute. Therefore, your experiences will vary.

The main thing is for you to try to raise your mind above the ordinary, concrete concepts of everyday life. If you can at least do this, you are doing well. Most people never put themselves into a situation where they can meditate or be sensitive and aware. If attending an initiation gives you the chance to do so, you should take the best possible advantage of that situation. You are not looking for some extraordinary experience. In this twentieth century it is enough simply to try to experience tranquillity, bliss, and transcendence. Why do I say it is enough simply to try? Just compare the life you usually lead in your samsaric nest with what you are doing at an initiation. Eating and dancing can never compare with trying to develop your mind.

Some people say, "I have received this initiation, and you haven't." I don't believe in that kind of arrogance. Among Tibetans, among Westerners, who can say who has received what initiation? Only the individual concerned can tell what initiation has or has not been received. You cannot determine this for others. That is why I usually allow any sincere person to come to an initiation. I cannot tell whether others' minds are high or low; I cannot tell whether the initiation will be helpful for them or not. Be careful. Even though you might harbor the arrogant thought that you have received this or that initiation, can you be sure? You might have been there when the initiation was being given, but perhaps you received nothing.

If you go to an initiation with the right attitude and an open mind, I am sure that you will receive an extraordinary vibration. That is enough. You do not have to be super-intellectual and ask, "Why do we do this? How does it work? What are all those Tibetan things for? I'm not going to take the initiation until I understand all that." That's nonsense.

VERSE SEVEN

Consciously and unconsciously, without control, we break our vows and commitments, pushed by a force like that of a raging thunderstorm. We find it extremely difficult to stop ourselves from doing so. I think, in a way, that people who believe themselves to be very pure and holy may be more negative than those who recognize how impure they are. The former never make any effort to purify themselves with prostrations, retreats, and so forth, while the latter will practice strongly to purify their minds. The uncontrollable downpour of negativities, the breaking of vows and commitments, the feeling of being impure, and the hallucinated vision of the result, the Vajra Hells, are all dualistic and have to be purified. We offer the tsok with a request for blessings to perceive only purity.

OFFERING TO THE VAJRA MASTER

The "circle of pure offerings" in the title is called a circle because both male and female deities gather to offer the tsok. When there are either male or female deities alone we do not refer to the tsok as a circle. According to tantra, their coming together makes the offering far more powerful. The next line says that the nectar we offer is free of the dualistic appearance of subject and object.

The vajra master replies. Each time you taste the tsok it goes to your navel chakra, causing an inconceivably blissful explosion of tum-mo energy within your central channel.

OFFERING THE REMAINING TSOK

The protectors to whom we offer this are the external, internal, and secret protectors, and we ask them to help us practice Dharma in order to benefit others in as many different ways as possible.

18

Heruka Vajrasattva Tsok: The Second Commentary

I wrote the short text, *A Banquet of the Greatly Blissful Circle of Pure Offerings: An Antidote to the Vajra Hells*, because I thought that we needed a powerful way of purifying our negativities and that this would be a good method of doing so. Even though it's very short, this text covers the entire graduated path, from renunciation to the tantric experience of enlightenment.

In texts like the *Guru Puja*, the offering section comes first and the review of the graduated path to enlightenment follows at the end. Here I have tried to include the graduated path subjects in the tsok offering verses. Each verse contains some lam-rim subject because I thought this was a more direct means of communicating what our lives lack, what ruins them, and how we can improve them. We begin with guru yoga, then move on to the precious human rebirth, impermanence and death, renunciation, bodhicitta, sunyata, and tantra.

Also, Western Dharma students do a lot of pujas—the *Guru Puja*, Tara puja, *jor-chö,* and so forth—so I thought I'd write a new one for them to play with in case they were getting bored with the others. Not only that. Since the regular pujas are rather long, and in today's world we're always short of time, I kept this puja brief. It's easy to do, and it finishes quickly. Anyway, it's a product of my own fantasies.

Now, what does the term "vajra hells" mean? "Vajra" can be relative or absolute; here I am referring to the relative vajra, as in vajra and bell, the tantric implements we use. The word means indestructible, diamond-like. Diamonds are stronger than most other materials; it is hard to destroy a diamond. That's the connotation of "vajra." Is it possible that there could be an indestructible realm of misery? Well, that's a bit of poetic license, a slight exaggeration. There's no such thing as an unchangeable, permanent phenomenon. Nevertheless, when you've been miserable a long, long time you might feel, "I'm never going to get over this." For most of us, depression lasts only a few hours, but there are people who remain depressed for their entire lives. They certainly feel that their misery is endless. That's a vajra-hell-like experience. Anyway, vajra hell is just an expression; you should not take it literally.

THE MERIT FIELD

Normally when we make offerings, we visualize the object to whom we are making the offering—in this practice the object of offering is Guru Vajrasattva. We also visualize and meditate on the Vajrasattva mandala, where Guru Vajrasattva resides.

The first two lines of this verse are talking about the quality of the visualization that you make. It is a transformation of light. *De* means bliss, and *tong* means the universal reality of sunyata; *nyi-su* means without dualistic entity. The Vajrasattva mandala manifests from an appearance that has those qualities. This is actually quite profound. Old students may understand it, but new, mushroom students will probably find it a bit dream-like, a kind of spacey new concept.

Fundamentally, we all have a limited conception of both the nature of ourselves and that of the world in which we live. Furthermore, we lay an exaggerated projection on top of our already limited view of reality. We do not penetrate to the heart of reality, and we don't even touch the reality of the ground on which we stand. This is the human problem. We have no insight into either our inner or our outer reality.

We always say that we want to improve the quality of our lives, to have happy, joyful, profound, meaningful lives. We use all kinds of words to describe the perfect life we'd like to have. To lead a perfect life you have to understand how you see both your own nature and that of external phenomena. Whether or not you can do that will determine whether or not your life will be happy.

A mandala is a view of a total, or complete, world, in which you recognize the basic nature without any artificial projection, without hallucinating. Then you have flexibility, some kind of choice. Preconceived ideas and holding the dualistic notion of self-existence make your life impossible. When you visualize a mandala, you see everything—yourself and your environment—in the nature of bliss; you touch the fundamental reality of all existence. With that sort of recognition, or comprehension, you can eliminate depression and other miseries and enjoy your life.

Then a question might arise: "How can you say that everything is blissful? That I'm blissful, flowers are blissful, my friend is blissful? Some things are miserable; how can you say that they can be transformed into blissful objects?"

When you touch the fundamental nature, the ultimate reality, of any phenomenon whatsoever, there is pleasure. Everything that exists is capable of bringing pleasure into your mind. But you are narrow. Your mind has neurotic obsessions such as, "I only like things that are purple." For you, only purple things are objects of beauty. This sort of neurotic, dualistic, unrealistic way of thinking only gets you into trouble. But that's what we do all the time, isn't it?

Check what your mind considers to be beautiful. True beauty is everywhere. California is not the only place where there's pleasure and an attractive environment. Every place has a beauty of its own.

You can see that an object's ability to give bliss is not dependent on the object itself. From the scientific point of view, every object has a sort of common reality, a shared fundamental nature. This true nature is what is really beautiful; this is what really gives you satisfaction.

The way we interpret the beauty of an object—by its shape, color, and so forth—is too relative, too conventional. Such beauty is like a yo-yo: this morning I see a particular object as beautiful; this evening it looks ugly. I myself go up and down. That's the main trouble. We need to have a broad view of what constitutes a blissful object.

According to the philosophy and psychology of tantra, if you have the blissful wisdom that comprehends the fundamental nature, or true reality, of all existence, everything manifests as a blissful object. If you do not have that wisdom, objects alone cannot make you blissful. Human experience shows this to be true. When you are having a painful, miserable time, nothing you see will make you happy. If I show you something beautiful when you feel terrible, will it make you happy? No. There's no magnetic energy. Normally, subject and object sort of magnetize each other to produce an atmosphere of pleasure or pain. The qualities of life do not come from outside but from your own degree of satisfaction. If you have the quality of richness within you, everything external will satisfy you.

A happy, satisfied family life comes from people's minds, not their material possessions. You can see how the lives of many rich families in America are more disastrous than those of the poor. Perhaps you won't admit this because you're in America's corner! But I'm not taking a shot at America just because I'm a foreigner. When I come to America, I don't have any particular agenda; I just look to see what's going on. Perhaps I'm critical because I'm not involved in the American way of life; if I were, I probably wouldn't notice the things that I see.

If you are born into this society, it is very hard to see that possessions don't bring happiness because the emphasis here is always on how wealth does bring happiness. However, this attitude is the complete opposite of the truth. Unfortunately, American society has been built up on that false premise, so you just have to deal with it.

True satisfaction comes from within yourself. This does not mean that you have to give up your American pleasures. But whether or not American pleasures become pleasurable for you depends on your mind: American pleasures can make you miserable. If that happens it is your own fault, not that of American society.

The Buddhist attitude is, "I am responsible for the quality of my life. I am responsible for my own satisfaction." You cannot blame your father or your mother, your husband or your wife. That sort of fault-finding is endless. It is endless because it is illogical and is no way to solve problems. Materialists and capitalists have incredibly wrong ideas. From the Buddhist point of view, wrong ideas are the main cause of suffering.

Wrong ideas create negative karma, which results in suffering. What is a fundamentally wrong idea? Thinking, for example, "My pleasure and success depend upon other people," or "A higher standard of living and more material possessions will bring me satisfaction," or "Material objects are all I need to be happy." Such ideas are completely wrong. If you know how to think, it won't matter whether your standard of living is high, low, or medium—you will know how to enjoy yourself. That is the most important thing.

Visualize that in front of the Vajrasattva mandala, all of space is filled by magnificent objects of the five senses, greatly blissful objects of [Samantabhadra's] offerings, as it says in the fourth line of the first verse. Also, in Buddhist practice, offerings are made not only to buddhas and other holy beings but to all sentient beings as well. You should recognize the divinity within other people: their potential for enlightenment, or buddha-potential. In tantra we transform all beings into greatly joyful and magnificently appearing dakas and dakinis. In the greatly blissful space of non-duality, all sentient beings manifest as dakas and dakinis in various aspects: joyful, peaceful, powerful, wrathful; a whole variety of different but totally unified manifestations. We see them as the embodiment of unified method and wisdom, not as hungry ghosts or other emanations of misery. If you visualize miserable-looking objects, you'll feel miserable yourself—uncomfortable, somehow.

Therefore, it is important to transform the nature of the object you visualize into great bliss and to recognize its fundamental reality, thereby eliminating all dualistic concepts. You can also visualize and offer any sense object whatsoever. Most of us are psychologically hung up by miserly and limited thoughts, such as, "Oh, I don't have enough money to take a holiday," even when we do have enough. When you practice this tsok offering, you should visualize limitless objects of the senses, as beautiful, blissful, and inexhaustible as possible, and offer them to all—buddhas and sentient beings—without discrimination. We need this kind of training.

Usually we give things to only the people we like, and don't give anything to those we dislike. That's the Western way. At least in the East we have plenty of beggars to keep us oriented toward giving to strangers. Rich people come along and give away thousands of rupees to the poor. They're not the rich people's friends, are they? It's just that the environment encourages this sort of thing. So we *do* have some good things in the East! Some people think that the third world has nothing at all to offer: "They haven't even got the brains to get rich and be happy."

Of course, the United States has its poor people, too. There are many hungry people rummaging through others' garbage all the time, eating stuff that has been thrown out. You can see all this on television and in the big cities. The rich don't give to the poor, not because they can't afford to but because they don't like them. They just let them go hungry. I'm not talking politics or religion here; that's just how it is. This attitude is very bad. The selfish mind gives to those it likes and not to those it doesn't, irrespective of other people's needs. Our own need is the most important thing; after taking care of that, we give. That's samsara.

We should train our minds in generous and impartial giving. But giving doesn't mean just handing over cash or something. Don't think, "I myself am poor. How can I give?" Real giving is having a giving attitude. Not giving is the miserly attitude of "I don't want to give." That is just selfish.

Offering tsok is excellent training in overcoming such attitudes: all sentient beings are guests at your offering party, and you make extensive offerings to them all. It is essential to train our minds in this way if we want to be successful in both our Dharma practice and life itself.

BLESSING THE INNER OFFERINGS

Remember that the way to offer anything is to recognize the fundamental nature, or mode of existence, of whatever it is you are offering. This applies to the actual offerings you have placed on your altar and to the magnificent offerings you visualize filling all of space.

The vast subject of inner offering has been explained elsewhere, so I'm not going to spend much time on it here.[24] However, say you are offering a bowl of tea. Visualize in the space above the bowl the letters OM, AH, and HUM from below up. Radiant white light emanates from the OM throughout the ten directions of space, magnetically attracting the supreme qualities of the body of all enlightened beings, who have great wisdom, great love and compassion, and extremely joyful lives. These qualities return to the OM in the form of light and sink into it. The OM melts into blissful energy and dissolves into the tea.

Red light radiates from the AH invoking the pure speech of the supreme beings of the ten directions. This returns and sinks into the AH, which melts into blissful light energy and also dissolves into the tea. Similarly, blue light radiates from the HUM, invoking the divine wisdom, love, and compassion of the supreme beings of the ten directions. These enlightened qualities return to the HUM in the form of light. The HUM too dissolves into the tea.

You can bless anything you eat or drink in this way. When you eat and drink things into which you have put such concentrated thought, the energy communicates and agrees with your nervous system. There is a kind of harmony between your physical nervous system and your consciousness.

In the West we'll partake of just about anything, even if it's completely unfamiliar to us. We don't communicate with the things we eat or drink. Such substances coming into your nervous system can be very destructive. They may even cause cancer. This is what happens when you are unaware or ignorant of what you eat and drink. You might find it hard to believe, but the human body is like a flower, not like rock or concrete. Do you believe that the human body is as organic as a flower or not? When you over-fertilize a flower, what happens? It burns out. Organic things need balance. I really believe that in the West, besides there being a breakdown in human relationships, there is also a breakdown in the relationship between people, the food they eat, and the environment.

Perhaps I don't know what I'm talking about. You probably think that a mushroom monk like me must be dreaming when he tries to describe life in America. Well, I'm joking a little, but to some extent I really feel that people in modern industrialized nations have very little appreciation of the importance of the nature of their food and drink. They just gobble up whatever's put in front of them. If they don't like something, they'll just take whatever else they can get: "No, I don't like this; bring me some Coke. No, some Seven-Up! No, some ginger ale!" Everything gets mixed up. This can shock your body; your nervous system can't cope and will cry out in protest. You have to pay attention to the organic nature of your body. Be conscious of what you eat and drink. With insight you can develop a communicative relationship with the things that nourish you.

Now, getting back to the offerings. The objects of the five senses should be recognized as the five wisdoms in the appropriate colors and in their true nature of blissful non-duality. They energize great bliss and satisfaction within you. Recognizing this is very helpful for your development of great bliss.

PRESENTATION OF THE OFFERINGS AND MANTRA RECITATION

Next is a sort of request made to the guru, to whom you are making this offering. The blissful nectar, the perfect energy, in this verse is fundamental to the attainment of all realizations. It is also the yogis' and yoginis' pure vision and, therefore, beyond the view of ordinary beings. The offering is made for the guru to enjoy with his non-superstitious, greatly blissful wisdom. There's an implication here: when we enjoy sense pleasures, we are full of superstition, or wrong conceptions. When higher beings enjoy pleasures, they do not react to them with superstition.

What do I mean by superstition? It is like this: I see, for example, a flower, and gradually, I develop a relationship with it. I touch the flower, grasp at its color. I think how wonderful, how kind and generous it is; how it gives me great pleasure; how nothing else gives me such pleasure. The flower becomes my best friend. This attribution of fine qualities to the flower is superstition. I'm superimposing upon the relationship a lot of qualities that are not actually there.

This puts great pressure on the relationship; as soon as you start describing the flower as this, as that, and as the other, you are putting pressure on the relationship. Each time you see the flower as wonderful, beautiful, and gorgeous, you bind yourself tighter and tighter. The whole thing becomes a fantasy; the communication is not realistic. It is too superficial. Tension builds up, and instead of being loose and relaxed, you are tied in knots. That is superstition. Building fantasy relationships with people and objects in that way can only lead to trouble.

Buddhas and bodhisattvas, on the other hand, enjoy pleasures in a far more reasonable way. They don't have our superficial, conventional, exaggerated way of relating to them. They are more realistic; they touch the fundamental nature of reality. Their pleasures are more stable and subdued, and bring great love and peace. That's why the last line of this verse asks Guru Vajrasattva to enjoy the supreme nectar with greatly blissful, non-superstitious wisdom.

So you can see now that superstition is the mind that misleads you by exaggerating the qualities of objects, by seeing things that are not really there. Superstition is unrealistic and makes your life a fantasy. But if you clearly understand your relationship with others, just as it is, there's not too much tension between you. If you can overcome superstition, you will always be happy. That's why we have meditations to eliminate superstition: to make you healthy and to bring clean-clear awareness, so that you are not polluted or deluded.

Any relationship, whether it's pleasurable or miserable, is impermanent, transitory. We ourselves are transitory, so our relationships must necessarily be transitory. We have to accept this. I think it is especially important for Americans to understand the nature of relationships. Relationships between men and women, between friends, between whomever, are changing all the time. At the same time, people are miserable. It is change that causes misery; I hope you understand this. Everything changes, so of course your friendships will change. If you understand that relationships are transitory by nature, you won't feel any pressure; you'll have space to communicate, to let go. You'll see how changing relationships make you unhappy. But don't think that it is the changing object that makes you miserable. No! It is your unreasonable communication within the relationship that is the source of confusion.

When your closest companion dies, you cry and feel terribly depressed. You may even stay depressed for a long time. That is not useful. Death is death; death is natural; death is okay. You should accept it. Of course, I'm only talking intellectually here.

Enjoyment without superstition is very difficult. Buddhism says that you should have great enjoyment and a blissful life. What prevents you from having this experience? Superstition. Because of superstition you do not touch fundamental reality.

VERSE ONE

In space is the rainbow body of Vajrasattva. This is in the nature of your spiritual guide, your deity, the dakas and dakinis, and your Dharma protector. There is a kind of similarity between the way that Christians recognize God as the only God and our recognition of the essential nature of Vajrasattva as the one true liberator. In this verse we ask Vajrasattva to purify our hallucinated, superstitious delusion that Vajrasattva is not of the essence of the guru, the deity, the dakas and dakinis, and the protector. *Trül-nang* means hallucinating, deluded. Anyway, this is superstition; not understanding is superstition. We are hallucinating; we have to purify this hallucination. Offering all magnificent sense objects to Guru Vajrasattva, we request blessings, or inspiration, that simultaneously born, great blissful wisdom will grow in our hearts.

While making the offering, meditate on purifying the hallucinated, dualistic vision, or concept, that does not recognize the unity of those holy objects but sees them as separate. Then recite the Vajrasattva mantra using one of the three usual meditation techniques (yän-de, män-de, or phung-de) for purifying negativities. This eradicates all superstition and negative appearances in general, and the hallucinated, dualistic vision mentioned in this verse in particular.

This practice is very powerful because you meditate while making the offerings, saying the prayer, and reciting the mantra. This has a strong impact on your mind: "I am hallucinating when I do not recognize the unity of Vajrasattva, my guru, my deity, the dakas and dakinis, and my Dharma protector. They are of the one nature, but I see them as two. This is an hallucination, an appearance projected by my dualistic concepts. This is what I have to purify."

VERSE TWO

Our human lives are precious and most meaningful, but we ruin them, render them useless, through the contamination of our five sense consciousnesses' craving for and grasping at pleasurable objects. We ask Vajrasattva to purify the hallucinated, dualistic appearance that causes us to cling to sense objects, and we make offerings with a request for blessings and inspiration to abandon clinging to the worldly pleasures of this life.

I thought it important to describe how we ruin our perfect lives. Now, there is nothing physically wrong with us, and even if we are sick, we can usually still do things with our body, speech, and mind. But most of the time we are consumed by useless actions, doing things that have no meaning. Eating, sleeping, and defecating are not enough. What makes our human life meaningless? What destroys it? Our five sense perceptions. They are the main problem. There's no bright, powerful wisdom behind them, so they come to dominate and control our lives.

Blindly, we follow our sense perceptions. They tell us, "Ice cream is fantastic!" So we eat ice cream in order to find satisfaction. Then what happens? Most people who eat a lot of ice cream are miserable. They get fat and think that other people don't like them. It's probably not true, but that's the kind of fantasy we project.

Our five sense consciousnesses crave for and grasp at sense objects. They ruin our lives by making us narrow. We don't serve others, and our lives become meaningless, devoid of satisfaction, and unhappy. The cause of all this misery is our preoccupation with the sensory pleasures of this life. This obsession has to be purified.

For example, many of us meditate, and we've all had some meditation experiences, but those experiences have always disappeared, haven't they? You have some great experiences in retreat, but when you get back home, your old habits surface, and your meditation experiences vanish. I know people who have had great meditation experiences, but they were just flashes, like lightning; they didn't last. All that's left is a hungry ghost!

I have no doubt that you too have had meditation experiences, but why do you fall back into misery when you stop meditating? Why, when you're not meditating, does your precious human life become useless, meaningless? Why do you fall back into the same old garbage? Because you fail to understand that all this world's pleasurable phenomena are illusory. As long as you think they are real, you will continue to ruin your life in this way. You think things are real because you can touch them with your hand: you may feel something, but it's not reality.

We have all had glimpses of something worthwhile in meditation, but afterward we have fallen into our old habits, and those valuable experiences have disappeared. That is because we do not recognize all our sensory experiences as illusory. They are mere mental projections, but we build up a fantasy relationship around them. We do fantasize. Take this flower, for example. I close my eyes and grasp it, hang on to it; I won't let it go. If I left it alone, it would stay nice, but as I get more and more attached to it, I destroy it. We don't have to be like that. We can see and enjoy the flower but at the same time, recognize it as a fantasy, an optical illusion, as not really existing as it appears to our eye. Our eye sense is completely deluded. From the Buddhist point of view, you should have no confidence in what your sense perceptions tell you; no confidence that things really exist as they appear to your senses.

How do you eliminate your sense perceptions' craving for and grasping at sense pleasures? By recognizing that the objects that appear to your senses are hallucinations. You should realize that you're hallucinating, whether you have taken drugs or not. This is true. You do not understand just what appears to your senses. Thinking that the fantasy is real poisons your sense perception and ruins your life. That's the point.

Your life is up and down all the time. You can't just blame your karma for this. Your sense perception keeps making decisions, "Good, bad; I like this; I don't like that." These decisions do not come from something way in the background, like your karma. It is actually your eye sense that's at fault. It conjures up an optical illusion, and you base your decision on that. Do you really think that you should base your life decisions on what your eyes tell you, what your physical sense perceptions tell you?

Thus, from the Buddhist point of view, you cannot have real faith or confidence in what your senses perceive. You think that just because you can touch or smell something, it must be real, whereas if you can't touch or smell it, it's not—because "I don't feel it." It's the same thing with people who come to a Dharma center for a meditation course. While they are there, they feel that they are getting something worthwhile and gaining some control over their lives, but when they get back home, they lose it all. Why is that? Why is it that when you are meditating at a center, you feel that you are gaining something, that you are on the path to liberation, but after only one night back in your regular environment, your mind completely changes. Check that out. I think it means that you don't actually understand Dharma.

Also, when you come to a center for a meditation course, you have some sort of fantasy about the environment, and you grasp at it as real. When you leave this environment, its reality disappears and is replaced by that of your new location. Thus, the valuable things you gained at the center vanish, and you end up with the misery and unhappiness of your old habits. What you don't understand is that no matter where you are, at the Dharma center, downtown, or back home, whatever you perceive is illusory, a projection of your own mind. For example, both your old girlfriend and your new one are illusory. You didn't realize that your old girlfriend's appearance was illusory, so of course you don't see that that of your new one is illusory too.

If you can realize—really understand—that the Dharma center environment is illusory, and with intensive conscious awareness keep this recognition with you wherever you go, your experiences will be very different from what they normally are. Whether you are in the big city, at the beach, or in the Himalayas, you can maintain the same energy, stay in the same space.

Buddhism is very realistic in its description of human nature. I'm sure you've all heard that you shouldn't be judgmental, discriminating between good and bad, and so forth. Normally we'll say, "Oh, nirvana! Fantastic!" and grasp at it, or "Yeekh, samsara is terrible!" and try to push it out of our mind. We say, "My guru is fantastic, Dharma is so fantastic!" and "That person is so awful." All these judgments are based on our own superstitious mind's interpretation of our own deluded perceptions. We have to recognize that.

But it is not enough to be convinced of all this intellectually, either. It has to be experienced. Actually, you have already had enough experience—enough to break your heart! So Buddhism is dealing with life, with experience, and that's the way it shows you how to be healthy, how to have a healthy mind. You know how to talk to yourself when you start to get extreme.

Perhaps Buddhism is true only here, at Vajrapani Institute, and when you go to San Francisco, it will become untrue! Anyway, brief meditation experiences at Dharma centers are not enough. You have to maintain continuous awareness of the right view, wherever you are.

This verse, then, is talking about how we render our lives useless. Most of us would like our lives to be useful for ourselves and others. We all look for satisfaction in our lives. What makes our lives meaningless and dissatisfied is the mind that grasps at the pleasures of the senses and at their concrete, permanent appearance. We must completely abandon both these faults. If we want our lives to be happy and satisfied, we must be determined to eliminate these faults forever. In order to do this, we need to understand clean-clear that the way sense pleasures appear is illusory. Nothing is permanent and unchangeable. That is why many Buddhist texts emphasize renunciation of all objects of grasping. We don't know how to gain satisfaction from our relationship with pleasurable objects of the senses. Normally we exaggerate the good qualities of pleasurable sense objects. That's why I say we are hallucinating. Our judgment is not at all realistic.

When you understand the nature, or reality, of sense pleasures, you have the space to let go. Sense pleasures come and go. That's how it is, and you accept it. Because we grasp at pleasure with hallucinated concepts, every time it disappears we get shocked and feel miserable. That is unreasonable. So, we are hallucinating.

As long as your hallucinating mind keeps exaggerating the good qualities of a pleasurable object, there is no way that you will ever be really satisfied. Therefore, Buddhism emphasizes understanding pleasures as they are, by knowing the quality of their being. Then you have space. This makes you less emotional: when you have pleasure, it's okay; you recognize it as illusory. When you don't have pleasure, that's okay, too. It is only your concrete concepts' grasping at the pleasure that makes you confused, dissatisfied, and emotionally disturbed.

Keeping in mind the meaning of this verse, recite the Vajrasattva mantra. At the same time, do the three usual meditation techniques to purify your concrete concepts, hallucinated appearances, any impure energy associated with your physical nervous system, and the ignorance that is the foundation of all these problems. Deep within your psyche you might feel, "It's impossible to purify all my shortcomings, grasping, and selfish attitude. How can I ever get rid of all that?" Even though intellectually you might accept that purification works or that the Buddhist teachings are correct, deep inside you have doubts. Practice of the Vajrasattva meditation can also eradicate all those impure doubts by showing you the possibility of completely eradicating all negative energy and giving you the great inspiration to do so.

VERSE THREE

"...Please bless me to generate immaculate renunciation." Our lives begin in misery, and throughout their duration we keep adding more and more confusion. There has to be a reason for this, a cause for what in Buddhism we call karma. That cause is delusion. With delusion we create the karma to lead ourselves repeatedly into misery and confusion. We get caught in an almost indestructible trap of neurotic concepts and emotions. What is happening is explained by the words *tsül-min yi-je* in the verse. It means that you are imagining something that has nothing to do with either the relative or the absolute reality of the objects you perceive; something that is unrelated to the characteristic nature of phenomena. What you see is only your imagination.

On the basis of that imagination, you develop hallucinated, concrete concepts, the ego-grasping mind, and dualistic concepts. That's the way it starts. You build up an unreal fantasy of the object in your imagination, your concrete conceptions harden, and then you decide, "Yes. This is good; that is bad." You hold on intensively to what you have called good and build it up further. You build it up with intensive strength. It has a long evolution. You build up this, you build up that, you make certain determinations about things, and in that way you build your own doctrine, your own world, your own Mount Meru. Then, it becomes very difficult for someone to tell you that you are wrong. You have built up too strong a fantasy. From the beginning, all these fantasies are just your own experiences, but for you they are reality. From the Buddhist point of view, all sentient beings are trapped by their egotistic, permanent, dualistic concepts, which are based upon their unrealistic, imagined fantasies. That is how we all get caught in the net of samsara.

As far as reality is concerned, the deluded mind is extremely superficial. It may be mixed with a little relative truth, but most appearances are strongly deluded, strongly hallucinated. All deluded superstitious concepts are dualistic—obstacles to be purified.

Each time you recite the prayer, you have to think quite precisely about your own state of being, your own life situation. With strong understanding of your own experience, "How deluded I am; how I deceive myself dualistically. Everything I do in my life is superficial. Whether I'm dealing with my work or my friends, it is always with superstition, completely removed from reality. I always build up an unrealistic, imaginary fantasy of any sense object I perceive. This is how I trap myself in samsara." With this strong understanding, recite the mantra with the three purifying meditation techniques. In this way your purification becomes very powerful.

The reason that the purification becomes so powerful is that you single out the real obstacle to your discovering reality. Just to recognize this is some kind of realization; even this is very difficult to do. As soon as you recognize the actual troublemaker, you begin to change. There's a natural transformation. Many times our purification is complete nonsense because we have no idea of what exactly our problem is. When you have a clean-clear understanding of your problem, you can do your purifying meditation properly, and it becomes very strong. You become more realistic, more sincere. Sincerity is an important part of religion and has to come from understanding your own life situation, how your own samsara has developed, and how you attain nirvana. Then you become serious about your practice, and your appreciation of the Buddhadharma grows.

By recognizing your problems and knowing how to practice purification, you ask blessings to develop pure renunciation. You have to develop pure renunciation, whether you are ordained or lay, Buddhist or non-Buddhist.

What does it mean to renounce the world? Take Shakyamuni Buddha, for example. He left his kingdom and went into the jungle. We call that renunciation. He had the sun, the trees, and the earth all around him, and although he had left his wife and family behind, perhaps he had other pleasures there. Now, since Westerners dedicate their lives to the pursuit of pleasure, it is important to know what renunciation means. From the Buddhist point of view, everybody in the world needs renunciation. Without it, there is too much suffering; people become crazy, brokenhearted, and emotionally disturbed. Being renounced means becoming more reasonable through knowing the characteristic nature of pleasure and the objects of pleasure.

Before Shakyamuni Buddha renounced the royal life, he had visited the town and seen various manifestations of suffering: old age, sickness, and death. He realized that there was no reason to cling to the reputation of being king or to the pleasures of marriage. He was flexible. He saw that he was okay with these things, but also that he'd be just as okay without them. He knew he could live in the jungle and be just as happy and healthy as he was in the palace. Flexibility is the key: you are all right if you get pleasure, and you are all right if you don't. In this way, you become very easygoing.

We Westerners are not easygoing. When we miss out on pleasure, we are not at all easygoing. That means we don't have renunciation. Renunciation does not mean that you have to give up ice cream, but rather that if you get ice cream, you enjoy it in a reasonable way, and if you don't get ice cream, you are still all right. You don't have to scream at your parents or your husband or your wife. Just think, "Okay, I'm not going to get any ice cream today. I'll still be okay." That's all right. Of course, I'm just using ice cream as an example, but you can apply all of what I'm saying to any relationship with other people or things.

If you get the chance to enjoy something, then enjoy it as much as possible but in a reasonable way—with dignity and a refined, or transcendental, attitude. Enjoy that pleasure as it is, instead of with delusion, superstition, and fantasy. When you discover the "as it is" of things, everything gives you pleasure. That's true. I really believe it. When you touch reality, you find and appreciate beauty everywhere and get pleasure from whatever object you encounter.

When we are ruled by fantasy, we become very particular and put limits on beauty: "Only this is beautiful." That's when the trouble starts. You have a limited conception of beauty, a limited conception of pleasure, so you exaggerate the beauty of the objects that give you pleasure and build up an inventory of "favorite things." That way you get confused and suffer. You are not open to the true nature of things; you are closed.

Look at all the advertisements on TV. They show you only objects of obsession. The people who make these ads show only one kind of beauty. They never show you flowers, for example. Why not? Check it out; it's human psychology. Those advertisers know how our minds work.

Beauty is everywhere. It is very important that you touch reality and place a reasonable value on each object, value it for its unique beauty, its own proportion of energy, its own relative reality, and its own absolute reality. You need to understand these notions in order to be flexible with pleasurable objects.

You can see from this why Buddhism is considered to be a realistic religion, philosophy, or doctrine—whatever you want to call it. Who can reject or disagree with the fact that your misery, confusion, and dissatisfaction come from your own deluded mind? Obstacles are within you; superstition, fantasy, concepts, and imagination are within you. Those factors are the cause of all your suffering and confusion. Who can disagree? This is a very simple, scientific thing.

Many people are scared of Buddhism. "Oh, Buddhism means you have to renounce. The Buddha gave up his wife and child and went into the jungle. He was irresponsible, a bad example for our society." That's a complete misunderstanding. Renunciation doesn't mean just tossing something out. For instance, your body is always with you. From the abhidharma point of view, even Guru Shakyamuni's body was samsaric.

Take Milarepa, for example. He gave up everything, including his teacher, and went off into the mountains. We say he renounced samsara, but he still had to take his body with him. His body was samsaric, wasn't it? The nettles he ate to sustain it were a samsaric phenomenon. But he was easygoing, he had no problem. Meanwhile, we're all hung up grasping at sensory pleasures. The most important thing is that we understand the nature of sensory pleasures, from both the side of the subject and the side of the object. Be reasonable.

Even in the Theravada Vinaya it is explained that whether or not a monk or nun has broken a vow depends mainly on the mind, not on the object or the action. Each vow has certain conditions under which it can be broken: motivation, object, action, and completion. All these branches of an action must be present for it to be complete. The main thing is the motivation, how much you are grasping.

Proper renunciation requires you to understand the nature of reality. Without understanding reality, there's no way you can develop renunciation; once you understand it, renunciation comes. Simply pushing doesn't work. Renunciation means discovering a new, basic reality.

The logic for all this is in the lam-rim: there's no reason to crave sensory pleasures because they're so small, so transitory, so impermanent; you're only deceiving yourself by craving and clinging to objects that you mistakenly see as permanent. In the lam-rim, you deal with reality, and reality talks to you. That helps release the pressure created by your grasping mind. I'm only talking theoretically, but if, in your everyday life, you analyze how your imagination builds up fantasies, how these fantasies become concrete, and how this leads to deluded action, you will understand the evolution of samsara through your own experience.

Maybe you're confused by the process of the Vajrasattva practice. On the one hand, we're asking Vajrasattva for the realization of renunciation, and on the other, we're offering him blissful sense objects.

If you ask people what their particular interests are, everybody will tell you something different. Some people like music, some art, others astronomy. That is wrong. In my opinion, each person should enjoy everything. Everybody should appreciate forms, colors, tastes, smells, and sounds; every sense object has the ability to give pleasure.

Therefore, it is good for you to offer all objects of the five senses to Vajrasattva, using your imagination as much as you can. Every phenomenon has its own beauty; beauty is a universal phenomenon. When you make your offering as extensive and beautiful as possible, you awaken the totality of your own mind to appreciate pleasure. We are so limited. Our minds cannot embrace the totality of pleasure. I do believe that within us we have the potential to experience complete pleasure, complete happiness, but we have to awaken it.

Why do some people like only certain objects and not others? You are capable of enjoying them all. You simply have to discover the total pleasure and satisfaction that are already within you. Don't complain, "I have such little pleasure. Everybody around me is miserable. I am miserable too." That is ridiculous. Just look around the world. There are so many different conditions, so many poor countries, so many people. But everybody finds some beauty, some pleasure, some purpose in life. Check it out. This is human experience, a scientific fact, not just religious dogma. In my opinion, even if you are depressed or upset, no matter where you are, you always have pleasurable objects with you.

Tantra talks about absolute beauty, but so far I've just been discussing relative beauty. Absolute beauty is sunyata, and tantra identifies it as female. This is simply a psychological expression. What you should try to understand is that beauty is limitless.

Try to discover relative beauty. We haven't even done that yet. With a partial mind we decide that one person, one little thing is the most beautiful of all. That's so limited. Try to discover the totality of both relative and absolute beauty. Then true renunciation will come. Is all this clear? Renunciation and offering all sense objects transformed into bliss go together. That is my message.

Sometimes renunciation means that you literally *do* have to give some things up. If you live in a big city and are trapped in a very disturbing situation, it may be hard to find space. In that case it is better to leave the situation for a while until your confused mind has had a chance to clear itself. That is important, because here the situation itself is making things difficult for you. You are not leaving because you are really renounced but because you are overloaded, overwhelmed, and without the space to sort out the mess. When you leave such a situation for a while, you can look at it objectively and see more clearly what to do. If you stay, day by day the confusion will build until it completely suffocates you. There's no way that wisdom can grow while you are smothered by the demon of dualistic conceptions. Therefore, it is important to go away for a while, but be skillful when you do so.

Real renunciation comes from understanding; simply moving away is not true renunciation. Many people already do this; when trouble comes, they go somewhere else. That's our style. Even the idea of a holiday is that you get away from your usual problems. You mean well, but it's not true renunciation. On the other hand, many Buddhist meditators have done the same thing, going to secluded places to escape from samsaric situations. It depends upon how you manage your life, how you cope with normal situations.

Remember the story of Lama Je Tsong Khapa? He studied and taught for years and had thousands of disciples. One day he selected eight bodhisattva-disciples and took them to a mountain retreat, where they remained isolated for a long time. It wasn't that he had to worry about samsara—he was already renounced—but through his actions he was telling us something: if you want to shift from your present level of consciousness to a higher one, you need a long period of peaceful tranquillity to practice intensive awareness.

That's why I always recommend that every year my students spend at least ten days in retreat, renouncing all their worldly relationships for a period of strong meditation. Cutting off completely for ten days is not too much, but at least it will give you a taste of renunciation. If you don't experience the peace and tranquillity of at least this level of renunciation, it will have no reality for you, and you won't be convinced of its benefits; renunciation will be just something else that you've heard of.

Experience is the most important thing. That's how you find solutions to your problems. Our problems—as mentioned in this verse—are so deeply rooted in our unconscious that it takes tremendous energy to eradicate them. It's certainly not a short, one-time job.

VERSE FOUR

Here we request inspiration to develop immaculate bodhicitta. "Bodhi" means totality; "citta" means heart. "Totality heart" implies that at present our hearts are narrow, not fully developed. What we have to change is our feeling that we ourselves are more dear than others. We have to get rid of this in order to open our hearts completely.

Why are we bored, lonely, and lazy? Because we don't have the will to totally open our hearts to others. If you have the strength of will to open your heart to others, you will eliminate laziness, selfishness, and loneliness. Actually, the reason you get lonely is that you are not doing anything. If you were busy, you wouldn't have time to get lonely. Loneliness can only enter an inactive mind. If your mind is dull and your body inactive, then you get lonely. Basically, this comes from a selfish attitude, concern for yourself alone. That is the cause of loneliness, laziness, and a closed heart.

There is no way to get everlasting satisfaction unless you change your attitude from one of holding yourself dear to one where you open your heart and dedicate yourself to others. If you can do this, you are guaranteed of satisfaction and will never be lazy.

The selfish mind is incredible, worse than a knife in your heart. Selfishness kills you, destroys your life. All the political troubles in the world today come from the selfish attitude. It doesn't matter what the object of your selfishness is—your own reputation, your own nation, the planet's resources, money—the selfish attitude is the main trouble-maker. We kill each other because of the self-cherishing thought, holding ourselves dear and not worrying about the welfare of others. All bad relationships—between husband and wife, guru and disciple—come from the selfish attitude. When you think about it, you can see that every problem on earth comes from being concerned for oneself instead of others.

Selfishness is painful, really painful. If you want to be free of the pain in your heart, open it by developing universal concern for others, bringing all sentient beings into your heart as much as you possibly can. That is the antidote to the selfish attitude that is the pain in your heart. I truly believe that this is the way to liberation.

We are always concerned that we won't be liberated. We don't want to be unhappy or emotionally disturbed; we want good relationships; we worry about our own welfare. We constantly talk about these things. The most practical way to liberate yourself from pain and emotion is to dedicate yourself to others as much as you can. This automatically eliminates the self-cherishing thought and the pain of selfishness. If you can't dedicate yourself to others, even equalizing yourself with them will stop the pain in your heart. Think, "I want to be as happy as possible; I don't want the slightest unhappiness. Others are the same. Irrespective of race, skin color, or anything else, in this we are the same. Therefore, I should not make myself uncomfortable by discriminating."

Trying to develop this attitude is easier than trying to develop indestructible meditation. It is powerful, easy to understand intellectually, and you already have a certain degree of this dedicated attitude within you. You just have to increase it. Also, meditators can become hypersensitive and full of anger. They don't want any distractions and can become quite selfish. Somebody makes a little noise, and they get upset: "You destroyed my meditation!" A practice that you can understand philosophically, psychologically, and scientifically can be a lot easier for you. "Others are most precious; I will dedicate myself to their welfare." The moment you dedicate yourself to others, you have space—the space not to get angry when somebody else abuses you.

I think most people do have a good heart and some dedication to others, but most of them are not meditators. That's why I feel that the dedicated attitude is so simple, so logical. It brings you an entirely different kind of satisfaction from what you normally experience and eliminates all kinds of negative thoughts. If you can adopt it, you'll be able to say that your dedicated attitude is your meditation, your life; your practice of awareness will be to eliminate your selfish attitude and dedicate yourself to others. If anyone can say this, I think it is wonderful. It is very practical if you can lead your life for the benefit of others. You may not become famous, but just to do it your own way is enough.

My parents used to disagree with each other over how to help others. My mother was a very practical person. Whenever an opportunity to help others arose, she took it. My father would tell her she was wrong; that she had to be selective in whom she helped. Her logic was, as she would tell my father, "Suppose you are travelling in some far off place and have no food and nowhere to stay. You ask some people for help but they tell you that you are not a worthy object of charity. How would you feel? No matter who comes to you, I think you should just serve them." In a way, they were both right, but my mother was more practical.

I don't need to go into the details of how to meditate on bodhicitta because it's all in the lam-rim teachings. Just remember that the attachment that holds yourself dearest of all is the cause of all misery. All the difficulties in the world—power struggles, the pursuit of wealth, hunger, fighting—come from cherishing oneself above all others. This is the problem, has always been the problem, and will continue to be the problem. Therefore, dedicate yourself to others as much as you possibly can. This is the only way you'll be happy—I think I can make that statement—nothing else can truly satisfy you. You don't have to be wealthy to dedicate yourself to others. Even if you have nothing, you can still dedicate your life that way.

So, I hope you are clear about all this. This verse refers to the door to all misery and confusion, which is self-cherishing, and to the demon, or chief evil, of dualistic conception, which is the mind that puts yourself first and others second. We offer transcendental, blissful sense objects to Guru Vajrasattva with a request to purify our dualistic concepts and appearances and to bless us to generate immaculate bodhicitta, the essence of the bodhisattva path. We're all trying our best to tread this path, but it's not easy. If you think you are a bodhisattva, check to see what a bodhisattva really is.

VERSE FIVE

This verse deals with sunyata, the great seal of emptiness (*mahamudra*). Historically, seals were used as signs of official approval; a seal held some kind of reality. "Seal of emptiness" might look a bit strange to you: "The seal is empty; empty means nothing. How could that do a good job? Why call it a seal?" From the Buddhist point of view, the state of non-duality is supreme. What does it hold? It embraces every existent phenomenon, without exception; non-duality pervades all existence, both relative and absolute.

We all look different: he, she, you, me, that, this. The person who understands non-duality sees the unity that lies beneath our different appearances. When we look at each other, we all seem so real, discrete, unconnected. The person who has realized emptiness sees us individually, but also as a whole, as if we were droplets in a cloud of steam. That is the seal. It holds the totality of absolute nature, just as it is. With a prayer for the understanding of the great seal to grow within us, we offer Guru Vajrasattva the blissful experience of the objects of the five senses.

All phenomena exist merely as images of mental speculation. You create some appearance and then proceed to label it, to give words to that reality. *Tok-pä par-zhak* means produced, or projected, by superstition. And all these things exist merely by imputation of name. There is not the slightest trace of self-existence in any phenomenon. Whatever you consider beautiful, ugly, wonderful, tasty, aromatic, or anything, it is simply a projection of your superstitious mind.

Advertising works because of this. Products are presented as excellent, successful, certain to make us happy, and so forth; ads make us believe that a particular product is worthwhile. As a result, we grasp at what we see as a self-existent object. First, it is nothing; then, the advertisers visualize, imagine, and fantasize; finally, they decide how to present it. Of course, the object does have its own relative and absolute function, but we grasp at it as self-existent. We're not aware of the evolution of superstitious projections.

Not that it is easy to understand this evolution. You need to think about it deeply and, in the light of that reflection, examine your everyday life so that you can gain some experience of how it works. You cannot understand it through just the words. You have to reflect on the fact that all existent phenomena, like things you consider useful or pleasurable, have no intrinsic value until you give them a name. Superstition applies a mental label, then their value appears. Until then they have no reality for you. That's why advertisers work so hard to make products real for you. In a way, they're very kind. But your responsibility is to realize that whatever they show you is a dualistic projection of the superstitious mind, and that you are only dreaming if you try to achieve absolute happiness through such objects. That sort of understanding is very helpful in relieving the pressure of your conceptualizing, grasping, egotistic mind.

To summarize, all existence is merely labeled, given value by superstition. This contaminated, foul-smelling (*dri-ma ngän-päi)*, dualistic hallucination has to be purified.

Each verse of this practice covers a different subject. You need to think about each one very deeply and intensively to know clearly what you should extinguish and what you should accomplish. From this clear understanding you will develop the strong motivation to purify the faults mentioned in the verse. Then you recite the Vajrasattva mantra with the three different meditation techniques. If you can practice like this, your purification will be logically based and, therefore, very sincere and extremely powerful.

Now, instead of my talking more, let's practice a short meditation. Think as follows. Two or three hundred years ago, none of the mentally labeled objects that we find today in supermarkets existed. Then, people started intellectualizing, and superstitious fantasies grew. Then, they produced Coca-Cola and all the other supermarket things with which we're so familiar. All these things have been labeled, or produced, by the mind of superstition. From their own side, these objects have no trace of duality or self-existence. As long as you want to see things dualistically, the dual appearance is there. When you see totality, dualistic appearances vanish. You and I are one totality of non-duality. Be aware of totality; feel totality. Totality has no idea of good or bad, beautiful or ugly. Now meditate on totality with intensive awareness.

Previously we were talking about the great seal of emptiness. Buddhism believes that all human beings have the ability to understand our own true nature, and that developing such understanding is the most important thing we can do. All the problems, confusion, and dissatisfaction we experience are the result of not having developed this understanding, and until we do, we shall never be free from bondage. The main human problem is not understanding our own reality.

Therefore, all the teachings of the Buddha, no matter which you choose, are directed at helping us realize both the conventional nature of our lives and universal totality, or sunyata. Both are of great importance.

So this fifth verse is referring to the Buddhist scientific theory of reality, describing first of all the conventional—relative or interdependent—way in which our body and mind exist. As our mind perceives these conventional existences, it tries to identify the reality of what it sees, to comprehend the reality of our own existence, others' existence, universal existence, the existence of all phenomena. And how do we end up? By *naming* perceived objects in an attempt to give them reality.

That's what *tok-pä par-zhak* means: something is there—a nectarine, for example—and what we try to do is identify its reality. So we give it the name "nectarine" to represent its reality. As a matter of fact, the true reality of the nectarine is just the collection of its constantly moving parts: the right elements have gathered, the fruit has developed organically, and it's somehow ready to eat. Apart from this superficial interdependence and moment-to-moment transformation of the elements that constitute the nectarine, you can't add further dimensions to its existence; to do so is to exaggerate, or what I call overestimate, its qualities.

When we understand the cooperative, interdependent mode of existence of the nectarine, its transitory energy, its color and vibration, and also the relationship between ourselves and the nectarine, we will begin to understand its universal reality—or at the least, we will have the potential to do so soon.

The first thing we have to realize—and this is important—is the way the conventional I, or self, exists; how it operates. If you investigate this, you will find that it exists simply by the mind's applying a temporary label to a bubble-like collection of parts: "It is that-this." The combination of the name and the bubble constitutes the conventional reality of the object. Apart from that, there is no absolute conventional reality: it is merely conventional.

Similarly, whenever you see a beautiful body, remember that it is simply an interdependent conglomeration of vibrations named by the mind. If you can understand conventional reality in this way, you will eliminate your habitual exaggeration and diminution of the relative truth. This is Buddhism's middle way, the way to eliminate confusion and become healthy. It is done by touching reality, comprehending the true nature of your own mode of existence. This is the door to satisfaction. From the Buddhist point of view, if you don't understand the true nature of conventional reality, you are only dreaming if you even talk about comprehending absolute truth; there's no way you can do it.

That's why Buddhist teachings always start with an explanation of the human dilemma: What is a human being? What qualities do humans possess? What problems do they face? Buddhist philosophy, psychology, and doctrine all deal with human reality: How do we eradicate all our problems? In other words, how do we become enlightened or, in philosophical terms, unify with the totality of being, as taught in the completion stage of tantra?

Lately I've developed a taste for nectarines. The other day Åge, one of my students, took me nectarine shopping, and we agreed that we should pick out only the good ones. So, we both selected some. Last night Åge and I were eating nectarines, and one of his was rotten inside. He said, "I picked this one; I thought it was okay, but it's rotten." He admitted it himself without my saying anything!

I'm telling this story because it's a good example of what we do. We pick something up, touch it, look at it closely, and finally declare, "Ah, here's a good one." But by the time we get home, it's rotten. Now, the question is—we've labelled a particular substance "nectarine"—but what is the reality of that substance? Is a rotten nectarine a nectarine?

Calling something a nectarine is supposed to somehow touch its reality, but from the Buddhist point of view this is a very superficial exercise. The superficial mind labels something a nectarine, and a nectarine comes into existence. But in our delusion, we hear the word nectarine and a concrete nectarine enters our perception. But there's no such thing as a concrete nectarine—inherently existent, independent, permanent. Fundamentally, the relationship between the name nectarine and the reality of the nectarine is for us the product of ignorance, developed through our not having touched the nectarine's reality.

Instead of thinking of a nectarine as a nectarine, try calling it "John"!

Give it a human name! We have a fixed idea about the name John. If I ask you why he's called John, what qualities did he have to warrant being called John, what are you going to say? Your answer will be very superficial; it won't even cover his beard! The name John doesn't even cover his beard. It might just cover a tiny part of his reality, but even that's doubtful.

Buddhism considers it very important that you don't jump to fixed conclusions, "You *are* John; I know you are." Instead, look at the history of that projection, why he was given that name. Then you can see how untrue it is that he really is John. Names are given to things and people in a very false way and have little to do with the reality of the named objects. Look at the history of conventional existences and you'll see why Buddhism says *tok-pä par-zhak:* the superficial, superstitious mind makes a certain projection, gives a name, and behold, a functioning human being. That's all it takes to make us function. We are so sure we know what we are. How can we be so sure when we choose rotten nectarines believing them to be good ones?

From the Buddhist point of view, human existence is the most sophisticated, most profound form of life—much harder to know than a nectarine. It is hard to understand who we are, what we are, and the true nature of both our relative and absolute modes of existence. But it is most worthwhile to develop this understanding.

Lord Buddha himself said, "I tell some disciples that things truly exist some others that things do not truly exist. I explain things differently according to the situation. It might look like I'm contradicting myself, but whatever I teach is to lead those particular disciples to a better understanding of reality. Therefore, don't necessarily believe something just because I said it." Everything Lord Buddha taught was to help us discover the two levels of truth: the relative and absolute truths of our own mode of existence. All his teachings were for this purpose.

How to stop delusion? First, recognize that the deluded mind is, in fact, deluded, that its concepts are false. Recognizing delusions for what they are is the only way to break them down.Therefore, you have to take responsibility for your own mind, analyze it, check it out thoroughly, in order to eliminate your confusion.

Recently I heard that some scientists are likening the brain to a camera. Of course, by "brain" they're referring to what we call consciousness.

But they come to the same conclusion as we do. They say the brain takes pictures of a certain vibration, but the reality of that entity is something else. I find that very interesting. Their description is the same as Lord Buddha's: conventional existence is nothing other than a gathering of interdependent energies. There is no permanent, concrete existence out there waiting for us. We always feel, and Westerners especially, that "out there," some wonderful companion is waiting for us. Perhaps that's why we find reality so difficult.

Another favorite example of mine is the linear accelerator. They take millions of photographs of a particle accelerating through the same space under completely controlled conditions, trying to get identical photographs, but every one turns out different. Why? Because they are filming an impermanent, relative phenomenon subject to conditions. It doesn't matter how many pictures they take—it's their thinking that's off track. We are so coarse that we can't see even the conventional movement of the process of change. This example shows how deluded our conceptions and sense perceptions really are.

In my opinion, just thinking about how your body exists, how your friend exists, is one of the best kinds of meditation. It makes you scared; instead of grasping at your friend you're afraid of him. You can even see him as a skeleton. That's the best way to eliminate your anxiety, grasping, and egocentricity.

Most people misunderstand the meaning of meditation. They think it's something that makes you numb. Meditation helps you overcome the distractions of the polluted, hallucinating mind and bring it closer to reality. I think that's what meditation should be. Lama Je Tsong Khapa said there were two kinds of meditation: analytical and single-pointed. It's possible that we're all meditating right now. We're intellectualizing, but even so, our minds have entered some kind of spiritual zone.

Now, I'd better get back to the text. All these prayers keep mentioning duality: duality this, duality that. Our mind is constantly dealing with conventional phenomena, so we are always in conflict. Don't think that by "conflict" I mean some kind of emotional disturbance. There are degrees of conflict; some conflicts are greater than others. As our mind operates on the basis of conventional phenomena, consciously and unconsciously, there are always at least two things in conflict. Our mind is always comparing one thing with another. All this is duality in action.

Nothing can exist for us unless we're comparing two things. Your not getting a job, things like that, everything is dualistic. But don't think that only the good-bad dichotomy is dualistic. Good itself can be dualistic: what you think of as good is usually just a fantasy. All the phenomena that you consider good and bad function dualistically because they are all relative, and even when you experience pleasure, it's dualistic, because it is limited. Your pleasure is limited because you function within the framework of duality. If you dismantle this framework, you will experience limitless joy.

VERSE SIX

The subject of this verse is tantra. I'm going to take for granted that you know from your previous tantric studies what the gross and subtle bodies and minds are.[25]

One of our biggest human problems is that we have a limited concept of ourselves. In other words, we put ourselves down. We have a low opinion of ourselves and a low opinion of others. "He did this, therefore, he is bad"; "I did this, therefore, I am bad." That kind of thing. We constantly see ourselves in a very ugly light; we project ourselves in an ordinary way. These are the problems that tantra can solve.

Ta-mäl nang-zhen means ordinary vision, ordinary projection, the generation of ordinary concepts. The way we appear to this ordinary mind and our very ordinary conceptions of ourselves are dangerous. They give rise to a limited, self-pitying image. All this prevents us from developing our human potential, from generating great love and great wisdom, from growing the totality of wisdom and love. If you project yourself as a limited, self-pitying entity, you become one because you believe, "I am this." You manifest like that. Tantra is the antidote to such ordinary, self-pitying ego conceptions.

To eliminate all this, you manifest in the present time the archetypal image of the deity, which gives you a self-image with divine qualities and a pure nature. This reflects your true mode of existence. Thus, you knock out the totally deluded, nonsensical, self-pitying image that your ego projects.

To do this properly you need strong penetrative insight and intensive awareness to convince yourself that you have the perfect qualities of a buddha or deity. You have to identify yourself in this way. Tantric practice is based on visualizing yourself as a deity and concentrating on that with divine pride.

The tantric method of eliminating the gross mind is to bring out the function of the subtle, unconscious mind by using such meditation techniques as the tum-mo or vase meditations. These techniques are designed to energize the fundamental consciousness that resides within the unconscious; to make it function at the conscious level. The gross mind has to be eliminated, because it is so deluded that it is a major obstacle to your touching reality. That is why you have to meditate.

Nyi-dzin lung-shuk drak-pöi. The gross mind is like a tornado because it shakes your life. Your dualistic mind shakes and disturbs your life. Our lives have been captured by the dualistic, superstitious mind. So my dualistic, superstitious mind brings me to California, then pushes me to Europe, then to Asia, and so forth. It always leads me here and there, driving me like a tornado. Maybe I'm exaggerating; check it out for yourself. The superstitious mind is very powerful; it makes all your life decisions for you.

Perhaps I can put this another way—I can say that your original mind is asleep; your fundamental mind is sleeping. It's as if it is closed for business and not taking any responsibility for your life. Who is taking that responsibility? Your superficial mind. That joker, your superficial mind, has taken over and is making all your life decisions. That's not fair. But if you can make yourself tranquil and peaceful, calm and clear, through practicing tantra, you can get your original mind to function. When it enters your central channel, you are automatically in contact with your own universal reality. We call that the clear light experience, or the vision of totality.

Why do we pray to attain the four actual initiations? Receiving initiations has more to do with your own level of development than with the guru's being something special. You don't receive an initiation just because the guru is special—in fact, it's the other way around; it's because of your own qualities. Because of your own mind's capacity to attain higher states, during an initiation it can somehow meet, or merge with, the guru's mind, such that you both experience the same thing. That sort of experience can really be called receiving an initiation.

If you happen to be in a place where an initiation is being given, you do receive something, of course, but probably not the real thing. *Nge-dön* means "that which can truly be defined as an initiation." Is that what you received? Did you experience the true nature of the relative initiation? It's all a question of your level of mind.

In ancient times, when highly qualified gurus gave initiations, some of their disciples would receive realizations instantly! Those sound like Western realizations—like instant coffee! But really, we know from history that the moment those highly qualified gurus gave the initiation, the mature disciple was magnetically opened, as if struck by a nuclear missile. The initiation would go straight into the disciple's heart, and he would be totally transformed. It's good to know these things. Usually, it's like what we're doing here: I sit up here talking nonsense; you don't touch reality while I talk; and of course, as soon as I go, you're going to forget everything I said anyway. Compared with the ancients, we're very poor quality practitioners. I guess I shouldn't say that about you, but it's certainly true for me.

People interpret the experiences of others very unrealistically. Let me give you an example. Say that I've explained a certain practice and that later a student comes to me to report having had a particular experience. I reply, "I don't believe you. You're just a mushroom student; you haven't studied Buddhist philosophy for twenty years. How can you claim to have had that experience?" Of course, I'm free to believe that his experience has no basis in reality and that without academic study one cannot touch reality, but I'd be wrong. How can I tell what someone else's level of consciousness is? You never know.

For a start, there is not only one life. We bring to our present life the experiences of countless previous lives. How can I pass judgment on someone else: "You haven't studied doctrine for a long time; you're a non-Buddhist from an irreligious country; you can't possibly have had an experience like that." But I don't know what's going on in that person's mind. How can I deny his experiences? Yet we deny other people's experiences, others' reality, all the time. That's not right; be careful. You cannot put others down.

Actually, all human experiences are transitory, momentary, impermanent, not inherently existent. Therefore, what you receive during an initiation depends entirely upon your own level of development. However, don't start thinking, "Oh, I've been to a hundred initiations—maybe I haven't received anything. It's all been a complete waste of time." That's not true. You must have received something—how much simply depends upon your own level of mind. The four great initiations have different stages; there are degrees of readiness for an initiation. There is no question that good things must have happened, but the real question is, did you receive the *actual* initiation?

Be reasonable; accept your own physical and mental qualities: "I'm all right. My face is not so horrible that I can't show it in my local supermarket. I've nothing to worry about." As soon as you start accepting yourself as you are, you begin to transform. Feeling good about yourself is itself some kind of transformation. In a reasonable way, bring your good qualities to mind and try to develop a positive attitude to life. With this as your foundation you will be more successful, more positive, and more realistic. This will lead to spiritual growth. It's a very practical way to be.

If you have a bad opinion of yourself, it's not a true picture, and you're only making your own life difficult.

VERSE SEVEN

We have so many negative imprints on our consciousness. We create them day by day, week by week, month by month. Why? Because our minds are uncontrolled. The more uncontrolled our minds and habits, the more we hallucinate and become deluded. The more we hallucinate, the greater the dark shadow of ignorance in our minds. The greater the dark shadow, the less the wisdom. Then fear and tension tend to arise, because everything is unclear. We are in the dark; our surroundings are murky. Neurotically, we project all our doubt, fear, unease, and anxiety into the darkness: "Maybe this is happening; maybe that is happening." We live in a world of fantasy, where fantasized reactions are the only reality, and this is how we end up in the vajra hells—a self-created hallucination of a dark prison. That, actually, is what the hells and the other miserable realms are.

There is no miserable place waiting for you, sitting and waiting like Alaska—waiting to turn you into ice cream. But whatever you call it—hell or the suffering realms—it is something that you enter by creating a world of neurotic fantasy and believing it to be real. It sounds simple, but that's exactly what happens.

So when you touch the really deep, deep, neurotic, hallucinated, deluded dark shadows, it is difficult to be calm and difficult to return from or go beyond that space. You can analyze this and see for yourself that it's true.

For example, many depressed people can be seen on American TV explaining how they've been depressed for so many years. You see, I don't need to go to some laboratory to do research; my TV set tells me exactly what's going on in your minds! Hell, or whatever you call it, has to do with your own mind and your own interpretation of reality. Whatever you interpret as reality manifests to you as reality.

Therefore, in this verse we pray for the infinite pure land to appear: *Dak-pa rap-jam ba-zhik char-war shok!* Psychologically, how does this work? If you have a completely positive attitude about yourself and touch the pure nature of your fundamental reality, your negative projections disappear, and the world improves. Your environment becomes positive, more beautiful, and attractive. So instead of projecting a dangerous world beset by pollution, radiation, and poisoned resources, you project an incredibly beautiful landscape of trees and water and gentle human beings all helping one another, which gives you great pleasure. If you can interpret the world in that way, it really will become a pure land for you.

So, the actual pure land depends a lot on your own mind. If your mind is happy, clean-clear, and in touch with fundamental reality, then the true nature of the pure land appears around you. When you have the pure vision in this life, you are guaranteed that it will continue in the next. That is the way that karma works.

The reverse, of course, is also true. If you are miserable, thinking ill of yourself and others and always emitting negative vibrations, the karmic impact of this experience guarantees that you will be reborn in a miserable place. Such a result is no more than the karmic impact of your own experience.

OFFERING TO THE VAJRA MASTER

With the next verse, the tsok is offered to the vajra teacher. It asks him to listen and to please enjoy the blissful nectar that is free from the confusion of dualistic concepts, which is offered by the courageous males and females, the dakas and dakinis.

Tantra understands that at the fundamental core of human existence lies inseparably united male and female energy. Practicing the path, we recognize the simultaneous existence of these energies. When we become enlightened, we manifest as Vajradhara, the total union of male and female. It is very important to know this.

In the perfect tantric gathering, men and women come to make offerings together. *Tsok-kyi khor-lo* means circle of offerings. It's called a circle because of the sense of unity or completeness of energies when men and women make offerings together. The totality of the experience is beneficial for each others' minds.

We usually enjoy things with a dualistic mind, but through tantra it is possible for us to enjoy sense objects non-dualistically.

In the next verse, the teacher replies, saying something like, "Oh, great blissful wisdom, the great collection of tum-mo heat energy; the experience is beyond words or concepts. Enjoy that great bliss forever." I don't need to say any more about this.

OFFERINGS AND PRAISE TO VAJRASATTVA; EIGHT-LEGGED PRAISE; SONG OF THE SPRING QUEEN

I don't need to say anything about these verses either. I didn't write them; they come from other practices. I'm sure you can find commentaries on them elsewhere.

OFFERING THE REMAINING TSOK

Earlier, we made offerings to the higher beings. Here, we offer to those who are lower. In Buddhist practice, we make offerings to all universal living beings. This is the path of training the mind. Your objects of charity should not be only higher beings. You should give something to everybody: to the buddhas and bodhisattvas, and to animals and other ordinary beings. Everybody is an object of charity.

Furthermore, even though we mean well, our concepts are usually so limited that most of the time we don't know what true charity really is. True charity is giving without ego, being true to your original nature. Remember, we are reflections of each other.

So we offer the leftover tsok in a skull cup as the illusory appearance of great bliss and emptiness united, recognizing that energy as the five divine wisdoms. We offer it to the positive worldly beings, those who help our spiritual growth in the four ways: peaceful, wrathful, developing, and controlling.

CONCLUDING PRAYER OF AUSPICIOUSNESS

These verses are also from elsewhere. I don't need to comment on them.

CONCLUSION

You can now see the extent of tantra's concern that the unity of your own male and female energies functions within you. The meditation techniques in tantra ensure that these two energies develop within your nervous system and energize your consciousness.

From the Tibetan Buddhist point of view, tantra is the final path. Lord Buddha gave many different teachings on various aspects of method and wisdom, but the highest of all was tantra. It shows that men and women are equal when it comes to attaining totality; they can unify the same realizations at the same time and in the same space; they can equally gain everlasting satisfaction. That's what Buddhist tantra explains.

We have to recognize that both men and women reflect each other. We have equal responsibility to gain the same realizations, reach the same destination, develop the same intensive awareness. We also have equal capacity to lead each other: women have the capacity to lead men to the highest destination, and men have the capacity to lead women to the same place. In particular, tantric theory shows clearly that without the help of women, men cannot achieve enlightenment. All the texts say so.

Everybody knows that the Geluk tradition is supposed to be very strict. The Geluk tradition comes from Lama Je Tsong Khapa, who was a monk. He once said that during one of his meditation retreats, at first, many ordinary women would come into his cave, but later, as his meditations progressed, real transformations of Vajrayogini would enter. The implication of this is that because he had given initiations to immature disciples, he experienced the negative result of visions of ordinary women instead of dakinis, but that as time went by, he purified that view.

What all this shows is that although Lama Tsong Khapa's tradition is very strict—and because of our mad elephant mind, we do need it to be strict—when we reach a certain point, when we give up and let go, everything comes to us just naturally. I think this is what Lama Tsong Khapa is saying. When he had completely purified himself of all negative imprints, the divine wisdom female was always there.

Milarepa and many other great meditators and saints also had some connection with females. Nagarjuna, for example, had a close relationship with Tara, as did many others. Those female aspects led them to many realizations. Similarly, we all need the help of female practitioners, directly and indirectly, inwardly and outwardly. It is only because of gross misconceptions that men and women put each other down.

When we talk about totality, we are not talking about something superficial; what women can do, what women can't do. We are talking about the potential for total development. In this, there is total equality between men and women. And the dakas and dakinis of tantra are also equally realized, having reached the same level of consciousness and attained the same realizations in order to help each other.

Tantra not only explains in detail the inner qualities of mind that must be realized but also certain female physical characterisitics that are important in the practice of tantra and how these female organs are energized. You can research all this later; I'd only bore you if I went into detail now.

It is important to recognize that when men and women gather together for tsok, it is more than physical. We gather for the infinite progression of human consciousness that eventually leads to total satisfaction. That motivation should be remembered in everyday life, and if it is, men and women will constantly be learning and getting support from each other.

Many great saints among the Tibetan lineage gurus were women, and we take refuge in them. When I first went to Europe, where there are many churches, I watched to see what the people were doing. I noticed the strong connection that Westerners seemed to have with the Virgin Mary. In European churches their devotion is so strong that they seem to offer more candles to her than they do to Jesus. My guess is that when they pray to the Virgin Mary, they feel an organic, heart-to-heart communication with her because of her form. This is simply human experience.

The devotion of Tibetan Buddhists to Tara results from a similar attraction. Not only serious practitioners but even businessmen feel it. They do Tara pujas for success in business. There is definitely something special about her.

The success of Buddhism coming to Tibet was due in large part to women. Tibet's first Dharma king, Songtsen Gampo, was converted to Buddhism by his Nepalese and Chinese wives, whom we regard as emanations of Tara. The king felt that without them, Buddhadharma could not have become perfectly established in Tibet.

This does not apply only in Tibet. Anywhere in the world, even in the political sphere, men cannot succeed without the support of women. There is a lot of evidence for this—you can see for yourselves.

Men and women can live harmoniously and help each other, not just in the temporal sense, but in the attainment of total satisfaction. You have to know this.

The main point is that your impurities are your own projection, your own symptoms. *You* are the one who created your self-image of "I am a bad person." Therefore, you are capable of overcoming this projection by practicing purification.

Now, this is my last talk here, and what can I say?[26] Certainly I would like to thank you all for sharing your pleasures with me; I have enjoyed my stay here very much. As you can see, I'm very healthy, so you should not worry. I'm happy and enjoying life. I would like to thank those people who have put so much energy into developing the facilities here at Vajrapani for the benefit of myself and others, and especially those who have worked so hard taking care of me like a baby. From my heart, thank you so much. I think that's all I can say.

Perhaps I can answer some questions. Are there any difficulties? Sometimes I produce more confusion than clarity, so please ask.

Q: Sometimes Buddhism says that good and evil are the same, and sometimes that good is better than evil. Which is it?

A: That's a good question. From the absolute, or ultimate, point of view, good and evil are the same, absolutely the same: when you experience totality, there is neither goodness nor evil in your consciousness. But relatively speaking, because your conventional mind interprets things as good and evil, they exist. It depends upon which level of mind you're speaking from. But I'd like to make another point here. If you have concrete conceptions of good and evil, you're in trouble. Lord Buddha taught that there is no concrete object of evil, no concrete object of good; both are non-dual, both are non-self-existent. They are made real only through the operation of dualistic conceptions.

From the practical point of view, knowing this can help you deal with everyday situations. When good things happen to you, it's not necessarily fantastically wonderful; when bad things happen, it's not a big disaster. So you can see how the good/bad dichotomy demonstrates the reality of our superficial mind. Good and bad are like a dream, nothing to get emotional about. Am I communicating with you or not? Practically, this knowledge is very important. Next time that you feel, "Oh, this is fantastic, excellent, genuine," when your mind projects so many superlative qualities on another person or some object, slow down, check it out more deeply. Try to realize that over-reacting to a beautiful object comes from a neurotic view of reality. This perspective keeps you psychologically stable and keeps your reality stable. If you exaggerate the good qualities of something, your mind is always up and down, soaring and plummeting, causing you so much disappointment. Be realistic, take the middle way: don't expect too much, don't reject too much. Enjoy your relationships in a reasonable way.

Q: Tantra is said to be the quickest path to enlightenment, but I've also heard it's the most dangerous. How do you know when you're ready to risk taking an initiation?

A: You and I, all of us, we're always speculating: "If I do this, maybe something good will happen; if I do that, maybe something bad will happen." Of course, it's true that we never know what's going to happen next; we don't know what's going to happen tomorrow. There are no guarantees. But as humans, we are always optimistic, speculating that something good is just around the corner.

Let's say that we're planning a trip to the beach to go swimming. We're expecting pleasure: sun, sand, sea—a peaceful day out. We also know that there could be danger—a hurricane, perhaps. That's also speculation. Nevertheless, we still go to the beach, expecting the best.

We go through a similar thought process when we consider taking an initiation. On the negative side, we know there's a great risk that we won't be able to keep the vows we take. But we also know that the benefits are limitless and that the energy we receive has great power. I remember His Holiness Song Rinpoche once saying that since you're going to hell anyway, you might as well take the initiation. He was always very direct. It is extremely important to practice tantra, so even if you're going to break the vows, it's better to take an initiation than not. Even if you're reborn in some miserable place, since the tantric imprints are on your consciousness, you'll eventually be reborn where you can practice it once again. Other lamas have said the same thing.

Furthermore, I don't consider the risky part, the breaking of vows, as a painful experience but rather as some kind of realization. Usually, we never test ourselves, we never put ourselves into testing situations. We just float about in the comfort zone. Until you are really psychologically free, you have to follow rules, or guidelines. But once you have attained liberation, you're free; you don't need those rules anymore. Having psychological rails makes it clear to you when you have crossed the boundary between constructive and destructive behavior. If you reach a point of difficulty you can ask yourself why? Is it because of your nose, your hands, your body? Or is it because of your mind? In this way, you can see that it's your mind that forces you off the rails.

Having boundaries also helps you estimate the amount of negative energy that forced you to break your vows. This is useful because it allows you to deduce how much positive energy you need to generate to neutralize that negativity. Tantra teaches that you can purify any negativity you can imagine. If you do twenty-one Vajrasattva mantras every day of your life, your mind will be extremely clean-clear. There is no negativity that the Vajrasattva mantra cannot purify. The science of this is very simple. When you break a vow, you generate a certain amount of negative energy; to counteract it, you need to generate an equal amount of positive energy in your mind.

Therefore, when you break a vow, encourage yourself: "I was responsible for that. I can purify it, too." This is the way to liberate yourself. Overcoming your own difficulties with your own skill makes you free. The main thing to remember is that negativities are transitory, conventional, interdependent phenomena. Instead of thinking unrealistically, "It's all my fault. I'm completely negative; I'll never be free," you can think, "I'm capable of creating negativities; I must be capable of purifying them."

Q: When you were talking about the inner offerings, you said that our indiscriminate consumption of food and drink shocks our nervous system. Could you please say more about that?

A: Physical sufferings, like cancer,are a result of our own mismanagement—unconsciousness of what our body needs and what we put into it. We are unrealistic. We don't understand our own organic nervous system: we have a low opinion of it, treat it very disrespectfully, and expect unreasonable things from it. We eat all sorts of things, many of which cannot be digested properly. I believe that all this damage to our nervous system causes cancer.

We have to develop a reasonable understanding of the organic nature of our physical being and treat it with respect. We should know what's appropriate according to time and space and should take the middle way, neither overloading our little body nor living an ascetic extreme.

Simply put, physical disorders come from a disorderly mind. We don't allow our body the time and space it needs to function properly, to digest and assimilate nutrients in a healthy way. We don't breathe properly, either. When we're miserable we hold our breath too long. We don't exhale fully, and our bodies get pumped up with retained air so that our nervous system can't function and our mind shakes uncontrollably. The result of all this is an unhealthy body. Remember the four foundations of mindfulness that the Buddha taught? One of those is mindfulness of the body. We are not mindful of our bodies, so we get sick.

I can probably go so far as to say that the more sophisticated the food produced by modern society, the sicker we get. Of course, there's cancer in India and Nepal, for example, but I think there's more of it in the West. I once saw one health expert, a doctor, report that there are diseases found in the industrial West that are rarely found in the third world, where life is more simple and natural. So I think it's obvious that we're expecting too much of our delicate nervous systems, telling them, "I want to eat this; you have no choice. Take it! Digest!" We can't survive like that. Our bodies are natural, organic phenomena—it's important to develop good eating habits. Food is medicine; it is much better for our health than the plastic, chemical drugs we usually think of as medicine.

Appendices

Appendix 1

The Yoga Method of the Glorious Supreme Heruka Vajrasattva

TAKING REFUGE

Sang-gyä chö-dang ge-dün-la
Tak-tu dak-ni kyab-su chi
Tek-pa sum-po tam-chä-dang
Näl-jor sang-ngak ka-dro-ma
Pa-wo pa-mo wang-lha-mo
Jang-chup-sem-pa dak-nyi che
Kyä-par-du-yang lop-pön-la
Tak-tu kyab-su chi-war gyi.

GENERATING BODHICITTA

Sem-chän kün-gyi dön-gyi chir
Dak-ni he-ru-kar gyur-nä
Sem-chän tam-chä he-ru-käi
Go-pang chok-la gö-par gyi.

[The vase meditation: The nine-round breathing exercise]

VISUALIZATION OF [HERUKA] VAJRASATTVA

Rang-gi chi-wor PAM-lä pä-ma-dang AH-lä da-wäi dän-gyi teng-du HUM-lä dor-je kar-po tse nga-pa te-wa-la HUM-gyi tsän-pa.

De-lä wo-zer trö. Dön-nyi jä. Dü yong-su gyur-pa-lä Dor-je Sem-pa kar-po.

The Yoga Method of the Glorious Supreme Heruka Vajrasattva[27]

Taking refuge

(Recite three times:)
Forever, I take refuge in Buddha, Dharma, and Sangha, and in the Sangha of the three vehicles, the dakas and dakinis of secret mantra yoga, the heroes and heroines, the gods and goddesses, the bodhisattvas and, in particular, my guru.

Generating bodhicitta

(Recite three times:)
I must become Heruka in order to lead all sentient beings to the sublime state of Heruka-hood.

[The vase meditation: The nine-round breathing exercise]

Visualization of [Heruka] Vajrasattva

Out of the void, about six inches above the crown of my head, appears the seed syllable PAM, which transforms into a thousand-petalled lotus. On top of the lotus appears the seed syllable AH, which transforms into a moon disc. In the center of the moon disc stands the seed syllable HUM. Suddenly, the HUM transforms into a white five-pronged vajra that has a HUM at its center. Much radiant light emanates from both the HUM and the vajra, going out into the ten directions and completing the two purposes. The whole universe melts into light. This light then returns to and is absorbed by the HUM in the vajra. The HUM and vajra also melt into light and transform into Heruka Vajrasattva.

Zhäl-chik chak-nyi. Dor-je-dang dril-bu dzin-pa. Dor-je kyil-trung-gi zhuk-pa. Yum Dor-je Nyem-ma kar-mo. Zhäl-chik chak-nyi. Dri-guk-dang tö-pa dzin-pä kyü-pa.

Nyi-ka-ang dar-dang rin-po-chei gyän na-tsok-pä trä-pa. Nyi-käi chi-wor OM drin-par AH tuk-kar HUM. Tuk-käi HUM-lä wö-zer trö-pä rang-dräi ye-she-pa chän drang.

OFFERING TO HERUKA VAJRASATTVA

OM KHANDA ROHI HUM HUM PHAT
OM SVABHAVA SHUDDAH SARVA DHARMA SVABHAVA SHUDDHO HAM

Tong-pa-nyi-du gy-ur. Tong-päi ngang-lä AH-lä tö-pa yang-shing gya-che-wäi nang-du sha nga dü-tsi nga-nam. Zhu-wa-lä jung-wäi ye-she-kyi dü-tsii gya-tso chen-por gyur.

OM AH HUM, HA HO HRIH

OM VAJRASATTVA ARGHAM PRATICCHA HUM SVAHA
OM VAJRASATTVA PADYAM PRATICCHA HUM SVAHA
OM VAJRASATTVA PUSHPE PRATICCHA HUM SVAHA
OM VAJRASATTVA DHUPE ARGHAM PRATICCHA HUM SVAHA
OM VAJRASATTVA ALOKE PRATICCHA HUM SVAHA
OM VAJRASATTVA GANDHE PRATICCHA HUM SVAHA
OM VAJRASATTVA NAIVEDYA PRATICCHA HUM SVAHA
OM VAJRASATTVA SHABDA PRATICCHA HUM SVAHA

JAH HUM BAM HOH
Nyi-su me-par gyur.

Vajrasattva is white. He has one face and two arms. He holds a vajra in his right hand and a bell in his left. He is sitting in the full lotus position with his hands in the embracing mudra. His consort, Dorje Nyemma, embraces him, her legs encircling his body. She is white and has one face and two arms. She holds a curved knife in her right hand and a skull cup in her left.

They are both dressed in robes of heavenly silk and adorned by precious jewel ornaments. [They both have seed syllables] OM at the crown chakra, AH at the throat chakra, and HUM at the heart. Brilliant light radiates from the HUM at the heart, invoking the divine supreme wisdom energy of all tathagatas.

OFFERING TO HERUKA VAJRASATTVA

OM KHANDA ROHI HUM HUM PHAT *(Cleanses the offerings)*
OM SVABHAVA SHUDDAH SARVA DHARMA SVABHAVA SHUDDHO HAM
(Purifies them)

All is void. A seed syllable AH appears out of the void. It turns into a huge white kapala containing the five meats and nectars. They melt, becoming an ocean of the amrita-energy of divine transcendental wisdom.

(Bless the offerings by saying three times:)
OM AH HUM HA HO HRI
(Offer them with:)
OM VAJRASATTVA ARGHAM PRATICCHA HUM SVAHA
(OM Vajrasattva, accept greeting water HUM SVAHA)
and similarly with PADYAM (foot-washing water), PUSHPE (flowers), DHUPE (incense), ALOKE (light), GANDHE (perfume), NAIVEDYA (food), and SHABDA (sound/music) *in place of ARGHAM.*

JAH HUM BAM HO
Become non-dual.

EMPOWERMENT BY THE BUDDHAS OF THE FIVE FAMILIES

Lar-yang tuk-käi HUM-lä wö-zer trö. Wang-gi lha-nam chän-drang.

OM PANCHA KULA SAPARIVARA ARGHAM....SHABDA PRATICCHA HUM SVAHA

"De-zhin-shek-pa tam-chä-kyi ngon-par wang-kur-du söl." Zhe söl-wa tap-pä de-nam-kyi ye-she-kyi dü-tsi gang-wäi bum-pa tok-nä OM SARVA TATHAGATA ABHISHEKATA SAMAYA SHRIYE HUM zhe wang kur.

Ku ye-she-kyi du tsi gang Mi-kyö-pä u gyän-ching.

Tuk-kar da-wäi teng-du HUM-gyi tar yi-ge gya-päi ngak-kyi kor-war gyur.

OFFERINGS TO HERUKA VAJRASATTVA

OM VAJRASATTVA ARGHAM...SHABDA PRATICCHA HUM SVAHA
OM VAJRASATTVA OM AH HUM

PRAISE

Nyi-me ye-she dro-wäi päl
Chok-tu mi-gyur de-wa che
Dik-tung ma-lü drung-jin-päi
Dor-je sem-chok-la chak-tsäl

MANDALA OFFERING

[Optional: long mandala]

OM VAJRA-BHUMI AH HUM! wang-chen ser-gyi sa-zhi/OM VAJRA-REKHE AH HUM! chi chak-ri kor-yuk-gi kor-wäi ü-su rii gyäl-po ri-rap/Shar lü-pak-

EMPOWERMENT BY THE BUDDHAS OF THE FIVE FAMILIES

Again, brilliant light radiates from the HUM at the divine heart, invoking all initiating deities of the five families.

(Make offerings to them with:)
OM PANCHA KULA SAPARIVARA ARGHAM...SHABDA PRATICCHA HUM SVAHA

"All tathagatas, please bestow on me the [Heruka Vajrasattva] initiation." Upon this request, all the tathagatas hold up their initiation vases, which are full of the amrita energy of divine transcendental wisdom, and the amrita starts to flow. As the mantra OM SARVA TATHAGATA ABHISHEKATA SAMAYA SHRIYE HUM is said, the initiation is conferred.

The divine body of perfect absolute wisdom, Heruka Vajrasattva, is completely filled by the amrita energy of blissful transcendental wisdom. Some amrita overflows and turns into Akshobhya, who adorns his crown.

The seed syllable HUM stands at the center of a moon disc at the divine heart, encircled by the one hundred syllable mantra [standing counterclockwise around the edge of the moon disc].

OFFERINGS TO HERUKA VAJRASATTVA

OM VAJRASATTVA ARGHAM...SHABDA PRATICCHA HUM SVAHA
OM VAJRASATTVA OM AH HUM

PRAISE

Non-dual divine wisdom, magnificent inner jewel ornament of all mother sentient beings; supreme, unchanging, everlasting great bliss; indestructible, magnificent wisdom mind that releases all sentient beings from all negativities of body, speech, and mind, especially broken vows and pledges: to you I prostrate.

MANDALA OFFERING

[Optional: long mandala]
OM Adamantine ground AH HUM! Mighty golden ground/OM Adamantine circumference AH HUM! Outside it is encircled by the circumferential wall,

po/Lho dzam-büi ling/Nup ba-lang-chö/Jang dra-mi-nyän/Lü-dang lü-pak/Nga-yap-dang nga-yap zhän/Yo-dän-dang lam-chok dro/Dra-mi-nyän-dang dra-mi-nyän-gyi da/Rin-po-chei ri-wo/Pak sam-gyi shing/Dö-jöi ba/Ma-mö-pa-yi lo-tok//Kor-lo rin-po-che/Nor-bu rin-po-che/Tsün-mo rin-po-che/Lön-po rin-po-che/Lang-po rin-po-che/Ta-chok rin-po-che/Mak-pön rin-po-che/Ter-chen pöi bum-pa/Gek-ma/Treng-wa-ma/Lu-ma/Gar-ma/Me-tok-ma/Duk-pö-ma/Nang-säl-ma/Dri-chap-ma/Nyi-ma/Da-wa/Rin-po-chei duk/Chok-lä nam-par gyäl-wäi gyäl-tsän/Ü-su lha-dang mi-yi päl-jor pün-sum-tsok-pa, ma-tsang-wa me-pa, tsang-zhing yi-du wong-wa/Di-dak drin-chen tsa-wa-dang gyü-par chä-päi päl-dän la-ma dam-pa-nam-dang/Kyä-par-du yang La-ma Dor-je Sem-pai lha-tsok-la zhing-kam ül-war gyi-wo/Tuk-je dro-wäi dön-du zhe-su söl//Zhe-nä dak-sok dro-wa mar-gyur nam-käi ta-dang nyam-päi sem-chän tam-chä-la tuk-tse-wa chen-pöi go-nä jin-gyi lap-tu söl!

[Optional: short mandala]
Sa-zhi pö-kyi juk-shing me-tok tram
Ri-rap ling-zhi nyi-dä gyän-pa di
Sang-gyä zhing-du mik-te ül-war gyi
Dro-kün nam-dak zhing-la chö-par-shok!

SECRET MANDALA

De-tong lhän-chik kye-päi ye-she-kyi
Zung-nam pung-kam kye-che-lä jung-wäi
Ri-ling rin-chen ter-bum nyi-dar chä
Kyab-gön tuk-jei ter-la ül-war gyi

in the center of which are Sumeru, King of Mountains/the eastern continent, Videha/the southern, Jambudvipa/the western, Godaniya/the northern, Kuru/[the eastern minor continents] Deha and Videha/[the southern] Camara and Apara-camara/[the western] Shatha and Uttara-mantrin/[and the northern] Kuru and Kauvara/[In the four continents are:] the precious mountain/the wish-granting tree/the wish-fulfilling cow/the unploughed harvest//[on the first level of Mount Sumeru:] the Precious Wheel/the Precious Jewel/the Precious Queen/the Precious Minister/the Precious Elephant/the Precious Horse/the Precious General/the Pot of Great Treasure/[on the second level: the eight goddesses,] Lady of Grace/Lady of Garlands/Lady of Song/Lady of Dance/Lady of Flowers/Lady of Incense/Lady of Lamps/Lady of Perfume/[on the third level:] the sun/the moon/the precious parasol/the banner of victory in all quarters/In the center, the most perfect riches of gods and human beings, with nothing missing, pure and delightful/To my glorious, holy, and most kind root and lineage gurus/and in particular to Guru Vajrasattva's deity host, I shall offer these as a buddha field//Please accept them with compassion for the sake of migrating beings. Having accepted them, to me and all migrating mother sentient beings as far as the limits of space, out of your great compassion, please grant your inspiration!

[Optional: short mandala]
This ground, anointed with perfume, strewn with flowers,
Adorned with Mount Meru, four continents, sun, and moon,
I offer in visualization as field of buddhas.
May all sentient beings thus enjoy this pure land.

SECRET MANDALA

The right view of sunyata is one with the wisdom of great bliss. This wisdom transforms into Mount Meru, the sun, the moon, and all other phenomena in the universe. I offer everything magnificent to you, ocean of great kindness, the one who is liberated and who liberates all others as well.

INNER MANDALA

Dak-gi chak-dang mong-sum kye-päi yül
Dra-nyen bar-sum lü-dang long-chö chä
Pang-pa me-par bül-gyi lek-zhe-nä
Duk-sum rang-sar dröl-war jin-gyi lop

IDAM GURU RATNA MANDALAKAM NIRYATAYAMI

PURIFICATION

Chom-dän-dä Dor-je Sem-pa dak-zhän sem-chän tam-chä-kyi dik-drip-dang dam tsik nyam-chak tam-chä jang-zhing dak-par dzä-du söl

Zhe söl-wa tap-pä tuk-käi ngak-treng HUM-dang chä-pa-lä wö-zer trö

Sem-chän tam-chä-kyi dik-drip jang sang-gyä sä-chä-la nye-päi chö-pa pül

De-nam-kyi ku-sung-tuk-kyi yön-tän tam-chä wö-kyi nam-par dü-nä ngak-treng HUM-dang chä-pa-la tim-pä de-lä dü-tsii gyün kar-po bap-pa yap-yum-gyi jor-tsam-nä bap

Rang-gi tsang-buk-nä zhuk-te lü tam-chä ye-she-kyi dü-tsii gyün-gyi gang

Go-sum-gyi dik-drip tam-chä sang-kyi dak-par gyur

MANTRA RECITATION

OM VAJRA HERUKA SAMAYAM ANUPALAYA. HERUKA TENOPATISHTHA. DRIDHO ME BHAVA, SUTOSHYO ME BHAVA, SUPOSHYO ME BHAVA, ANURAKTO ME BHAVA. SARVA SIDDHIM ME PRAYACCHA. SARVA KARMA SUCHA ME CHITTAM SHREYAH KURU, HUM! HA HA HA HA HOH! BHAGAVAN VAJRA HERUKA MA ME MUNCHA. HERUKA BHAVA MAHA SAMAYA SATTVA AH HUM PHAT!

OFFERING AND PRAISE

OM VAJRASATTVA ARGHAM...SHABDA PRATICCHA HUM SVAHA
OM VAJRASATTVA OM AH HUM

INNER MANDALA

Please bless me and all other sentient beings to be released immediately from the three poisons, for I am offering without the slightest hesitation or attachment all objects of my greed, hatred, and ignorance; friends, enemies, and strangers; and my body and all possessions. Please accept all this.

IDAM GURU RATNA MANDALAKAM NIRYATAYAMI

PURIFICATION

"Bhagawan Vajrasattva, please purify all negativities and broken and damaged pledges of myself and other sentient beings."

Because of this request, brilliant light radiates from the mantra rosary and the HUM at the divine heart. It purifies all negativities and obscurations of all sentient beings and becomes an offering for all buddhas and bodhisattvas. The essence of the perfect qualities of their holy body, speech, and mind returns in the form of light, which dissolves into the HUM and the mantra rosary.

[From the HUM and the mantra rosary] a stream of blissful white amrita energy begins to flow down through the chakras of the divine couple. It flows out through the chakra of union and enters my crown chakra. This stream of amrita of transcendental wisdom fills my whole body, destroying all the negativities and obscurations of my body, speech, and mind. These are completely purified.

MANTRA RECITATION

OM VAJRA HERUKA SAMAYAM ANUPALAYA. HERUKA TENOPATISHTHA. DRIDHO ME BHAVA, SUTOSHYO ME BHAVA, SUPOSHYO ME BHAVA, ANURAKTO ME BHAVA. SARVA SIDDHIM ME PRAYACCHA. SARVA KARMA SUCHA ME CHITTAM SHREYAH KURU, HUM! HA HA HA HA HOH! BHAGAVAN VAJRA HERUKA MA ME MUNCHA. HERUKA BHAVA MAHA SAMAYA SATTVA AH HUM PHAT!

OFFERINGS AND PRAISE

OM VAJRASATTVA ARGHAM...SHABDA PRATICCHA HUM SVAHA
OM VAJRASATTVA OM AH HUM

Nyi-me ye-she dro-wäi päl
Chok-tu mi-gyur de-wa che
Dik-tung ma-lü drung-jin-päi
Dor-je sem-chok chak-tsäl tö

REFUGE IN HERUKA VAJRASATTVA

Dak-ni mi-she mong-pa-yi
Dam-tsik-lä-ni gäl-zhing nyam
La-ma gön-pö kyap-dzö-chik!
Tso-wo dor-je dzin-pa-te
Tuk-je chen-pöi dak-nyi-chän
Dor-wäi tso-la dak kyap-chi

ABSORPTION

Dor-je Sem-päi zhäl-nä:
"Rik-kyi bu (or bu-mo) kyö-kyi dik-drip-dang dam-tsik nyam-chak tam-chä jang-zhing dak-gö"
Zhe sung-nä rang-la tim-pä rang-gi go-sum-dang Dor-je Sem-päi ku-sung-tuk yer mi che-par gyur

DEDICATION

Ge-wa di-yi nyur-du dak
Dor-je Sem-pa drup-gyur-nä
Dro-wa chik-kyang ma-lü-pa
Kye-kyi sa-la gö-par-shok!

Non-dual divine wisdom, magnificent inner jewel ornament of all mother sentient beings; supreme, unchanging, everlasting great bliss; indestructible, magnificent wisdom mind that releases all sentient beings from all negativities of body, speech, and mind, especially broken vows and pledges: to you I prostrate.

Refuge in Heruka Vajrasattva

Through ignorance and delusion, I have broken and damaged my pledges. Holy Guru, who has the power to liberate me, my inner master, holder of the vajra, whose essence is great compassion, Lord of all migratory beings, to you I go for refuge.

Absorption

Vajrasattva says, "Oh son (or daughter) of good family, your negativities and obscurations and damaged and broken pledges are cleansed and purified." Then he dissolves into me. My three doors (of body, speech, and mind) become inseparably one with Vajrasattva's holy body, speech, and mind.

Dedication

Because of this merit, may I quickly become Heruka Vajrasattva and lead each and every sentient being into his divine enlightened realm.

Colophon

Because of encouragement from many intelligent Westerners that there was a need for a text for the sadhana of Vajrasattva that eliminates hindrances and produces profit on the stages of the path and is a preliminary to meditation on the two stages [of highest yoga tantra], one called Muni Jnana [Thubten Yeshe] has written this as an emergency delusion-cutter, so he asks forgiveness.

Appendix 2

The Heruka Vajrasattva Tsok Offering

A Banquet of the Greatly Blissful Circle of Pure Offerings: An Antidote to the Vajra Hells

THE HERUKA VAJRASATTVA TSOK OFFERING

A Banquet of the Greatly Blissful Circle of Pure Offerings: An Antidote to the Vajra Hells

INTRODUCTION[28]

THE TANTRIC TEACHINGS of Shakyamuni Buddha state that meditation on Vajrasattva is a preliminary practice for the generation and completion stage meditations of highest yoga tantra. Furthermore, Vajrasattva meditation is necessary during the stages of the path themselves, in order to complete both collections of merit and wisdom, to remove the various blockages and interferences that arise at different points along the path, and to help you familiarize yourself with the successive realizations as they are gained.

In order to practice Vajrasattva, your mind must first be made suitable. This is accomplished by receiving the permissions (*je-nang*) of body, speech, mind, qualities, and divine action, which are similar to the four great initiations. After doing this, and abiding in either the extensive or the abridged yoga of this deity, you can begin the *Banquet of the Greatly Blissful Circle of Pure Offerings: An Antidote to the Vajra Hells*, and, as has been said, [you can truly say,] "I am a fortunate, blissful one." These permissions, which are of the highest yoga tantra aspect of Vajrasattva, have been transmitted through the ear-whispered lineage of the Geluk tradition of Tibetan Buddhism, and the warmth of the blessings of this lineage continues undiminished down to the present day. Therefore, this practice of Vajrasattva is available for you to practice, and you can do so secure in the knowledge that it is in no way mistaken.

What follows is a tsok offering ceremony specifically designed to be performed in conjunction with the highest yoga tantra aspect of Vajrasattva. The Tibetan term *tsok,* which is often left untranslated, literally means "collection," or "assembly," and in the following practice it is often rendered as "pure offerings." However, the actual tsok is one's meditation on transcendental, blissful wisdom. The entire purpose of offering the tsok ingredients is to generate the experience of this blissful wisdom within oneself and to overcome the ordinary appearance and conception of sensory objects. Thus, it is extremely important that from the very beginning of this practice you prevent ordinary appearances and conceptions from arising. Because the offering of tsok is a profound method for transcending mundane thought, the entire practice should go beyond your ordinary experience of subject and object.[29]

MEDITATION ON THE MANDALA OF GURU VAJRASATTVA: THE FIELD FOR THE COLLECTION OF MERIT

HUM!
De-tong nyi-su me-päi nam-röl-lä
Jung-wäi Dor-je Sem-päi zhäl-yä-kang
Ten-dang ten-päi kyil-kor yong-dzok dün
Kün-zang chö-trin nam-käi kyön-kün kang

Nyi-me de-wa chen-pöi ka-ying-la
Ngo-tsar dor-nam lha-dang lha-möi tr-ül
Zhi-gyä wang-drak trül-päi gar-kän-gyi
Tap-she yong-su dzok-päi kur zheng-gyur

BLESSING THE OFFERINGS

OM KHANDA ROHI HUM HUM PHAT

OM SVABHAVA SHUDDHA SARVA DHARMA SVABHAVA SHUDDHO HAM

Tong-pa nyi-du gyur tong-päi ngang-lä AH-lä tö-pa yang-zhing gya-chewäi nang-du sha nga dü-tsi nga-nam zhu-wa-lä jung-wäi ye-she-kyi dütsii gya-tso chen-por gyur

OM AH HUM HA HO HRI *(say three times)*

PRESENTING THE OFFERINGS AND RECITING THE MANTRA

Ta-mäl wang-pöi yül-lä rap-dä-shing
Yo-gäi dam-tsik dak-nang de-wa-che

PRELIMINARIES

Place on the altar clean and beautiful looking offerings as well as *bala* and *madana*.[30] After completing either the abbreviated or elaborate meditation on the generation of oneself in the form of Vajrasattva,[31] visualize as follows:

MEDITATION ON THE MANDALA OF GURU VAJRASATTVA: THE FIELD FOR THE COLLECTION OF MERIT

HUM!
In the space before me,
From the enjoyment of indivisible great bliss and emptiness,
Appear the complete supporting and supported mandalas of Vajrasattva.
Clouds of Samantabhadra's offerings fill all of space.

In the sphere of great non-dualistic bliss
All beings miraculously appear as gods and goddesses
Embodying thoroughly developed method and wisdom
As skillful dancers manifesting peace, expansion, power, and wrath.

BLESSING THE OFFERINGS

(The offering ingredients should then be blessed in the following manner by reciting:)
OM KHANDA ROHI HUM HUM PHAT
(All those who create obstacles are dispelled, and by reciting:)
OM SVABHAVA SHUDDHA SARVA DHARMA SVABHAVA SHUDDHO HAM
(they are purified of ordinary appearances. Then visualize:)

All becomes empty and from the sphere of emptiness
Appears the letter AH which transforms
Into a very large and spacious skull cup
Containing the five meats and five nectars.
Melting, they all transform into a great ocean of wisdom nectar.

OM AH HUM HA HO HRI *(say three times)*

PRESENTING THE OFFERINGS AND RECITING THE MANTRA

This pure offering is the yogi's commitment (samaya)
And, as the pure vision of their great bliss,

Ngö-drup kün-gyi zhir-gyur dü-tsii chok
Tok-me de-wa chen-pö nye-par dzö

1. HUM! Ka-ying ja-tsön Dor-je Sem-päi ku
La-ma yi-dam ka-dro chö-kyong-gi
Ngo-wor ma-tok nyi-dzin trül-nang dak
Dam-dzä dö-yön na-ngäi tsok-chö-la
La-ma Dor-je Sem-pa nye-chir bül
Lhän-kye de-chen kye-war jin-gyi-lop

OM VAJRA HERUKA SAMAYAM ANUPALAYA. HERUKA TENOPATISHTHA. DRIDHO ME BHAVA, SUTOSHYO ME BHAVA, SUPOSHYO ME BHAVA, ANURAKTO ME BHAVA. SARVA SIDDHIM ME PRAYACCHA. SARVA KARMA SUCHA ME CHITTAM SHREYAH KURU, HUM! HA HA HA HA HOH! BHAGAVAN VAJRA HERUKA MA ME MUNCHA. HERUKA BHAVA MAHA SAMAYA SATTVA AH HUM PHAT!

2. HUM! Ka-ying ja-tsön Dor-je Sem-päi ku
Dö-yön de-la chak-päi nam-she ngä
Däl-jor dön-me ja-wäi trül-nang dak
Dam-dzä dö-yön na-ngäi tsok-chö-la
La-ma Dor-je Sem-pa nye-chir bül
Tse-dii nang-zhen dok-par jin-gyi-lop
OM VAJRA HERUKA SAMAYAM....

Transcends being an object of ordinary senses.
It is the basis of all attainments and the most supreme nectar.
Therefore, O Guru, with your non-superstitious
Simultaneously born great bliss, please enjoy it!

1. HUM! O miraculous rainbow cloud
Appearing in the space of dharmakaya,
Holy body of Vajrasattva—
Having purified the hallucinated vision
And dualistic conception that fails to recognize
That the guru, in essence, is the deity,
The dakini, and the Dharma protector—
In order to please you, Guru Vajrasattva,
I am presenting these sacred ingredients
As pure offerings to be enjoyed by your five senses.
Please bless me to generate simultaneously born great bliss.[32]

OM VAJRA HERUKA SAMAYAM ANUPALAYA. HERUKA TENOPATISHTHA. DRIDHO ME BHAVA, SUTOSHYO ME BHAVA, SUPOSHYO ME BHAVA, ANURAKTO ME BHAVA. SARVA SIDDHIM ME PRAYACCHA. SARVA KARMA SUCHA ME CHITTAM SHREYAH KURU, HUM! HA HA HA HA HOH! BHAGAVAN VAJRA HERUKA MA ME MUNCHA. HERUKA BHAVA MAHA SAMAYA SATTVA AH HUM PHAT![33]

2. HUM! O miraculous rainbow cloud
Appearing in the space of dharmakaya,
Holy body of Vajrasattva—
Having purified the hallucinated vision
Of the five sense consciousnesses' clinging
To the pleasure of desirable objects,
Thereby depriving this perfect human birth of all meaning—
In order to please you, Guru Vajrasattva,
I am presenting these sacred ingredients
As pure offerings to be enjoyed by your five senses.
Please bless me to abandon clinging
To the ordinary concepts and appearances of this life.
OM VAJRA HERUKA SAMAYAM....

3. HUM! Ka-ying ja-tsön Dor-je Sem-päi ku
Tsül-min yi-je nam-tok lä-nyön-gyi
Drip-yok nyi-dzin dön-gyi trül-nang dak
Dam-dzä dö-yön na-ngäi tsok-chö-la
La-ma Dor-je Sem-pa nye-chir bül
Nge-jung nam-dak kye-war jin-gyi-lop
OM VAJRA HERUKA SAMAYAM....

4. HUM! Ka-ying ja-tsön Dor-je Sem-päi ku
Rang-nyi che-dzin duk-ngäl kün-gyi go
Nyi-dzin dü-kyi gong-pöi trül-nang dak
Dam-dzä dö-yön na-ngäi tsok-chö-la
La-ma Dor-je Sem-pa nye-chir bül
Nam-dak jang-sem kye-war jin-gyi-lop
OM VAJRA HERUKA SAMAYAM....

5. HUM! Ka-ying ja-tsön Dor-je Sem-päi ku
Tok-pä par-zhak ming-kyang tak-yö-la
Nyi-dzin dri-ma ngän-päi trül-nang dak
Dam-dzä dö-yön na-ngäi tsok-chö-la
La-ma Dor-je Sem-pa nye-chir bül
Chak-gya chen-po tok-par jin-gyi-lop
OM VAJRA HERUKA SAMAYAM....

3. HUM! O miraculous rainbow cloud
Appearing in the space of dharmakaya,
Holy body of Vajrasattva—
Having purified the hallucinated vision:
The demon dualistic conception and veiling obscurations
Of improper attention, superstition, karma, and delusions—
In order to please you, Guru Vajrasattva,
I am presenting these sacred ingredients
As pure offerings to be enjoyed by your five senses.
Please bless me to generate immaculate renunciation.
OM VAJRA HERUKA SAMAYAM....

4. HUM! O miraculous rainbow cloud
Appearing in the space of dharmakaya,
Holy body of Vajrasattva—
Having purified the hallucinated vision
Of holding oneself more dear than others:
The door to all suffering and the dualistic conception
That is the chief of all evils—
In order to please you, Guru Vajrasattva,
I am presenting these sacred ingredients
As pure offerings to be enjoyed by your five senses.
Please bless me to generate immaculate bodhicitta.
OM VAJRA HERUKA SAMAYAM....

5. HUM! O miraculous rainbow cloud
Appearing in the space of dharmakaya,
Holy body of Vajrasattva—
Having purified the hallucinated vision:
The stench of dualistic conception holding
What is merely imputed by superstition as true—
In order to please you, Guru Vajrasattva,
I am presenting these sacred ingredients
As pure offerings to be enjoyed by your five senses.
Please bless me to realize the great seal of emptiness.
OM VAJRA HERUKA SAMAYAM....

6. HUM! Ka-ying ja-tsön Dor-je Sem-päi ku
Ta-mäl nang-zhen kün-tok tra-rak-kyi
Nyi-dzin lung-shuk drak-pöi trül-nang dak
Dam-dzä ye-she nga-yi ts-ok-chö-la
La-ma Dor-je Sem-pa nye-chir bül
Nge-dön wang-zhi top-par jin-gyi-lop
OM VAJRA HERUKA SAMAYAM....

7. HUM! Ka-ying ja-tsön Dor-je Sem-päi ku
Nye-tung drak-char wang-me bap-pa-lä
Dor-je nyäl-wa nyong-wäi trül-nang dak
Dam-dzä yeshe nga-yi tsok-chö-la
La-ma Dor-je Sem-pa nye-chir bül
Dak-pa rap-jam ba-zhik char-war shok
OM VAJRA HERUKA SAMAYAM....

OFFERING TO THE VAJRA MASTER

Dor-je dzin-pa gong-su söl
Pa-wo pa-mo tsok-kor de
Zung-dang dzin-päi trö-pa dräl
Dü-tsii de-la tak-tu röl
A LA LA HO!

E-MA! De-chen ye-she, kyäi!
Tsok-chen tum-mo bar-wäi drö

6. HUM! O miraculous rainbow cloud
Appearing in the space of dharmakaya,
Holy body of Vajrasattva—
Having purified the hallucinated vision
Of ordinary appearance and conception:
The eighty superstitions both gross and subtle,
The violent, uncontrollable wind of the dualistic mind—
In order to please you, Guru Vajrasattva,
I am presenting these sacred ingredients
As pure offerings to be enjoyed by your five senses.
Please bless me to receive the four actual empowerments.
OM VAJRA HERUKA SAMAYAM....

7. HUM! O miraculous rainbow cloud
Appearing in the space of dharmakaya,
Holy body of Vajrasattva—
Having purified the hallucinated vision
Of experiencing the vajra hells
Resulting from the uncontrollable downpour
Of negative actions and broken samaya—
In order to please you, Guru Vajrasattva,
I am presenting these sacred ingredients
As pure offerings to be enjoyed by your five senses.
May infinite purity alone arise!
OM VAJRA HERUKA SAMAYAM....

OFFERING TO THE VAJRA MASTER

(The offering of tsok to the vajra master should now be made while reciting:)
O holder of the vajra, please pay attention to me!
This pure offering presented by the assembled circle of dakas and dakinis,
This nectar free of all divisions of subject and object,
Transcendentally blissful, please enjoy it eternally!
A LA LA HO!

(The vajra master then replies:)
O hail, great blissful wisdom!
The great collected offering,

Ma-sam jö-dä ga-de-la
Kün-kyang aho sukha che

AHO MAHA SUKHA HO!

OUTER AND INNER OFFERINGS TO VAJRASATTVA

OM GURU VAJRASATTVA SAPARIVARA ARGHAM...SHABDA PRATICCHA HUM SVAHA
OM GURU VAJRASATTVA SAPARIVARA OM AH HUM

VERSES OF PRAISE

Gang-gi tsän-tsam jö-pä kyang
Lä-ngän dik-tung ma-lü-pa
Kä-chik nyi-la drung-jin-päi
Dor-je Sem-pa-la chak tsäl

EIGHT-LEGGED PRAISE

OM Chom-dän pa-wöi wang-chuk-la chak-tsäl HUM HUM PHAT!
OM Käl-pa chen-pöi me-dang nyam-päi wö HUM HUM PHAT!
OM Räl-päi chö-pän mi-zä-pa-dang dän HUM HUM PHAT!
OM Che-wa nam-par tsik-pa jik-päi zhäl HUM HUM PHAT!
OM Tong-trak chak-ni bar-wäi wö-zer-chän HUM HUM PHAT!
OM Dra-ta zhak-seng dung-dang katwang dzin HUM HUM PHAT!
OM Tak-gi pak-päi na-za dzin-pa-chän HUM HUM PHAT!
OM Ku-chen dü-ka gek-tar-dzä-la dü HUM HUM PHAT!

OM Chom-dän-dä-ma dor-je pak-mo-la chak-tsäl HUM HUM PHAT!
OM Pak-ma rik-mäi wang-chuk kam-sum-gyi HUM HUM PHAT!
OM Jung-pöi jik-pa tam-chä dor-je chen-pö jom HUM HUM PHAT!
OM Dor-je dän-zhuk zhän-gyi mi-tup wang-je chän HUM HUM PHAT!

The seed that causes the tum-mo heat to explode,
This joyful, blissful experience beyond concepts, beyond words—
Welcome, great eternal bliss!
AHO MAHA SUKHA HO!

OUTER AND INNER OFFERINGS TO VAJRASATTVA

(The outer and inner offerings are then presented while reciting:)
OM GURU VAJRASATTVA SAPARIVARA ARGHAM...SHABDA PRATICCHA HUM SVAHA
OM GURU VAJRASATTVA SAPARIVARA OM AH HUM

VERSES OF PRAISE

(Praise is offered by reciting the following:)
Merely thinking of just your name
Eradicates all obstacles
And immediately purifies all negative karma.
Thus to you, unsurpassed Vajrasattva,
I pay homage and make prostration.

EIGHT-LEGGED PRAISE

(Next recite the following in praise of Heruka and Vajravarahi:)
OM I prostrate to the Bhagawan, lord of the brave ones HUM HUM PHAT!
OM To you whose brilliance equals the fire that ends a great eon HUM HUM PHAT!
OM To you who have an inexhaustible crowning top-knot HUM HUM PHAT!
OM To you with bared fangs and a wrathful face HUM HUM PHAT!
OM To you whose thousand arms blaze with light HUM HUM PHAT!
OM To you who hold an axe, uplifted noose, a spear, and skull-staff HUM HUM PHAT!
OM To you who wears a tiger-skin cloth HUM HUM PHAT!
OM I bow to you whose great smoke-coloured body ends all obstructions HUM HUM PHAT!

OM I prostrate to the Bhagawati, Vajravarahi HUM HUM PHAT!
OM To the queen of the female arya practitioners, invincible in the three realms HUM HUM PHAT!

OM Tum-mo tro-möi zuk-kyi tsang-pa kem-par dzä HUM HUM PHAT!
OM Dü-nam trak-ching kem-pä zhän-gyi chok-lä gyäl HUM HUM PHAT!
OM Muk-je reng-je mong-je kün-lä nam-par gyäl HUM HUM PHAT!
OM Dor-je pak-mo jor-je dö-wang-ma-la dü HUM HUM PHAT!

SONG OF THE SPRING QUEEN

1. HUM! De-zhin shek-pa tam-chä-dang
Pa-wo dang-ni näl-jor-ma
Ka-dro dang-ni ka-dro-ma
Kün-la dak-ni söl-wa-dep
De-wa chok-la gye-päi He-ru-ka
De-wä rap-nyö ma-la nyen-jä-nä
Cho-ga zhin-du long-chö-pa-yi ni
Lhän-kye de-wäi jor-wa-la zhuk-so
A-LA-LA! LA-LA HO! A! I! AH! ARA-LI HO!
Dri-me ka-dröi tsok-nam-kyi
Tse-wä zik-la lä-kün dzö

2. HUM! De-zhin shek-pa...söl-wa-dep
De-wa chen-pö yi-ni rap-kyö-pä
Lü-ni kün-tu yo-wäi gar-gyi-ni
Chak-gyäi pä-mar röl-päi de-wa che
Näl-jor-ma tsok-nam-la chö-par dzö
A-LA-LA! LA-LA HO! A! I! AH! ARA-LI HO!
Dri-me ka-dröi tsok-nam-kyi
Tse-wä zik-la lä-kün dzö

OM To you who destroy all fears of evil spirits with your great diamond-like means HUM HUM PHAT!

OM To you whose eyes empower those who sit upon the diamond throne not to be conquered by anyone HUM HUM PHAT!

OM To you whose wrathful body on inner fire can desiccate Brahma HUM HUM PHAT!

OM To you who terrify and dry up all demons and thus can vanquish all other forces HUM HUM PHAT!

OM To you who triumph over all that can make one ill-tempered, excited, or stupefied HUM HUM PHAT!

OM I bow down to Vajravahari, the consort who overpowers lust HUM HUM PHAT!

SONG OF THE SPRING QUEEN

(Here, the "Song of the Spring Queen" may be sung to request realizations:)

1. HUM! We make our requests to you,
The tathagatas who are thus gone,
As well as to the viras, yoginis, dakas, and dakinis.
Heruka, who enjoys great bliss,
Intoxicated with bliss brings satisfaction to the consort
And in accordance with the precepts of practice
Enters into the union of innate bliss.
A-LA-LA! LA-LA-HO! A! I! AH! ARA-LI HO!
You, the multitudes of immaculate dakinis,
Look upon us with love; bestow all the powerful attainments.

2. HUM! We make our requests…dakinis.
Through the stirring of the mind of great bliss
Through the moving dance of the body
There arises the great bliss played within the lotus of the consort.
This bliss we offer to the multitudes of yoginis.
A-LA-LA! LA-LA-HO! A! I! AH! ARA-LI HO!
You, the multitudes of immaculate dakinis,
Look upon us with love; bestow all the powerful attainments.

3. HUM! De-zhin shek-pa...söl-wa-dep
Yi-wong zhi-wäi nyam-kyi gar-dzä-ma
Rap-gye gön-po kyö-dang ka-dröi tsok
Dak-gi dün-du zhuk-te jin-lop-la
Lhän-kye de-chen dak-la tsäl-du söl
A-LA-LA! LA-LA HO! A! I! AH! ARA-LI HO!
Dri-me ka-dröi tsok-nam-kyi
Tse-wä zik-la lä-kün dzö

4. HUM! De-zhin shek-pa...söl-wa-dep
De-chen tar-päi tsän-nyi dän-pa kyö
De-chen pang-päi ka-tup du-ma-yi
Tse-chik dröl-war mi-zhe de-chen yang
Chu-kye chok-gi ü-na nä-pa yin
A-LA-LA! LA-LA HO! A! I! AH! ARA-LI HO!
Dri-me ka-dröi tsok-nam-kyi
Tse-wä zik-la lä-kün dzö

5. HUM! De-zhin shek-pa...söl-wa-dep
Dam-gyi ü-su kye-päi pä-ma zhin
Chak-lä kye-kyang chak-päi kyön ma-gö
Näl-jor-ma chok pä-mäi de-wa-yi
Si-päi ching-wa nyur-du dröl-war dzö
A-LA-LA! LA-LA HO! A! I! AH! ARA-LI HO!
Dri-me ka-dröi tsok-nam-kyi
Tse-wä zik-la lä-kün dzö

6. HUM! De-zhin shek-pa...söl-wa-dep
Drang-tsii jung-nä-nam-kyi drang-tsii chü
Bung-wäi tsok-kyi kün-nä tung-wa tar
Tsän-nyi druk-dän tso-kye gyä-pa-yi
Chu-ching-pa-yi ro-yi tsim-par dzö
A-LA-LA! LA-LA HO! A! I! AH! ARA-LI HO!
Dri-me ka-dröi tsok-nam-kyi
Tse-wä zik-la lä-kün dzö

3. HUM! We make our requests…dakinis.
Yoginis dance with enchanting, soothing movements
The protector so exceedingly to please,
And the multitudes of dakinis
Come before us and bless us.
Bestow upon us innate great bliss.
A-LA-LA! LA-LA-HO! A! I! AH! ARA-LI HO!
You, the multitudes of immaculate dakinis,
Look upon us with love; bestow all the powerful attainments.

4. HUM! We make our requests…dakinis.
The great bliss which is possessed of liberating qualities—
The great bliss without which freedom cannot be gained in one life
Though one endures many asceticisms—
That great bliss abides within the centre of the supreme lotus.
A-LA-LA! LA-LA-HO! A! I! AH! ARA-LI HO!
You, the multitudes of immaculate dakinis,
Look upon us with love; bestow all the powerful attainments.

5. HUM! We make our requests…dakinis.
As with a lotus born out of mud,
Great bliss, though born of desire is unstained by its faults.
O supreme yoginis, by the bliss of your lotus
May the bonds of samsara be quickly untied.
A-LA-LA! LA-LA-HO! A! I! AH! ARA-LI HO!
You, the multitudes of immaculate dakinis,
Look upon us with love; bestow all the powerful attainments.

6. HUM! We make our requests…dakinis.
Like a swarm of bees drawing forth the nectar of flowers
May we likewise be satiated
By the captivating nectar of the mature lotus
Possessed of six qualities.
A-LA-LA! LA-LA-HO! A! I! AH! ARA-LI HO!
You, the multitudes of immaculate dakinis,
Look upon us with love; bestow all the powerful attainments.

OFFERING THE REMAINING TSOK

OM AH HUM *(say three times)*

De-tong yer-me gyu-mäi ka-pa-lar
Ye-she nga-yi dü-tsii tsok-lhak-nam
Zhing-kyong drek-pa de-gyä tsok-la bül
Dam-chö drup-päi lä-zhii trin-lä dzö

CONCLUDING PRAYER OF AUSPICIOUSNESS

Pün-tsok ge-lek je-wäi trün-päi ku
Ta-yä dro-wäi re-wa kong-wäi sung
Dro-wäi sam-pa ji-zhin zik-päi tuk
Rang-sem la-mar jäl-wäi tra-shi shok

Jung-gyüi chi-war bar-do kye-wa sum
Jong-je ku-sum lam-du kyer-wäi tü
Rang-sem nyuk-sem tra-mo jäl-wa-lä
Ku-tuk zung-juk char-wäi tra-shi shok

Trö-dräl ka-ying tong-pa chen-pöi yum
Nang-si de-wa chen-pöi ye-she-la
Kyü-päi ya-tsän kor-dä ngö-po kün
De-tong chen-por dom-dzä tra-shi shok

OFFERING THE REMAINING TSOK

(Finally, the way to offer the remainder of the tsok is as follows:)
OM AH HUM *(say three times)*

To the assembly of the eight classes of wrathful governing protectors
I present all the remaining pure offerings—
The nectar of the five wisdoms contained in this skull cup—
An illusory appearance of indivisible bliss and emptiness.
Do your duty, the four rites for Dharma practitioners.

CONCLUDING PRAYER OF AUSPICIOUSNESS

May all be auspicious for me to see my mind as the lama:
Who understands perfectly all beings' thoughts,
Whose speech fulfills countless beings' wishes,
And whose pure body arises from an infinite collection of merit.

May all be auspicious for realizing the unity of dharmakaya and rupakaya
By discovering my own subtle, continually-residing consciousness
Through the power of taking the three bodies as the path:
The antidote to coming death, bardo, and rebirth.

May all be auspicious for everything within samsara and nirvana
To be synthesized with great emptiness and great bliss
Through the unusual embrace of the mother: the sphere of space
Beyond all puzzling divisions, and the father:
The great blissful wisdom, the appearance of all existent phenomena.

COLOPHON AND DEDICATION[34]

On the special day of the daka and dakinis—the twenty-fifth day of the eleventh month of the Iron Bird year (19 January, 1982)—Venerable Lama Thubten Yeshe wrote this tsok offering of Heruka Vajrasattva for a puja performed at Bodhgaya under the bodhi tree by an international gathering of sangha and lay students who together made hundreds and thousands of offerings. This puja was offered by the Italian gelong Thubten Dönyö, a disciple having unsurpassed understanding of the sutra and tantra path to enlightenment and indestructible devotion to Shakyamuni Buddha's teachings, and who is adorned outwardly with saffron robes and inwardly with the three sets of vows.

This tsok offering was written with the prayer that all the sangha of the ten directions enjoy harmonious relationships with one another, guard the precepts of pure moral conduct, and accomplish the practice of the three higher trainings, thereby becoming skillful guides providing great help to all beings. It is dedicated to the speedy return of our great guru of unmatched and inexpressible kindness, Kyabje Trijang Dorje Chang. For the benefit of all sentient beings, our mothers, may we remain inseparable from this great guru during our entire path to enlightenment.

Furthermore, it has been noted that in many countries today —Tibet, for example— those whose lives are *not* opposed to the three ordinations of the pratimoksha, bodhicitta, and tantric vows are not considered to be human beings! Yet even in such extremely degenerate times there are still many fortunate practitioners, and it is very important that these yogis and yoginis have a method, such as this Vajrasattva practice, powerful enough for achieving the exalted realization of simultaneously born great bliss and emptiness. This profound method is easy and simple to practice, accumulates a great store of meritorious potential, and is capable of destroying all the negativities resulting from breaking one's pledged commitments. In fact, it is such a powerful method that many lamas of the Geluk tradition have stated that even transgressions of root tantric vows can be purified by reciting the Vajrasattva mantra. Therefore, one should understand that there is no negativity so strong that it cannot be purified through the practice of Vajrasattva.

For all these reasons, then, this tsok offering has been composed by Vajrasattva yogi and follower of Guru Shakyamuni Buddha's teachings, the bhikshu Muni Jñana.[35]

POSTSCRIPT

The following poem in jest came uncontrollably and without premeditation to the mind of the author while he was composing this work:[36]

All of samsara appears
As a foe to one who fears
He might be gored and torn
By the proverbial rabbit's horn
Of tantric ordinations:
The golden ground foundation.

In the common path untrained,
In tantra unordained,
He has no initiation;
What a situation!
How strange! What a joke!
He's a sky-flower yogi!

This tsok offering can be made to other highest yoga tantra deities by substituting that deity's name for Vajrasattva's and by blessing the offerings in accordance with the yoga method of that deity and reciting that deity's mantra.

The above was translated with the kind assistance of Lama Thubten Zopa Rinpoche and Ven. Konchog Yeshe, and edited by Jonathan Landaw. The "Song of the Spring Queen" was adapted from a translation by Ven. Jampa Gendun and Andy White, and the praises to Heruka and Vajravarahi were adapted from a translation by Alexander Berzin.[37]

Appendix 3
Tibetan Texts

༡

༄༅། །དཔལ་མཆོག་རྡོ་རྗེ་སེམས་

དཔའི་རྣལ་འབྱོར་

བཞུགས་

སོ།།

༡

༄༅། །སྐྱབས་འགྲོ་སེམས་བསྐྱེད་ནི། སངས་རྒྱས་ཆོས་
དང་དགེ་འདུན་ལ། །རྟག་ཏུ་བདག་ནི་སྐྱབས་སུ་མཆི། །
ཐེག་པ་གསུམ་པོ་ཐམས་ཅད་དང་། །རྣལ་འབྱོར་གསང་
སྔགས་མཁའ་འགྲོ་མ། །དཔའ་བོ་དཔའ་མོ་དབང་ལྷ་
མོ༔ ༔བྱང་ཆུབ་སེམས་དཔའ་བདག་ཉིད་ཆེ། །ཁྱད་
པར་དུ་ཡང་སློབ་དཔོན་ལ། །རྟག་ཏུ་སྐྱབས་སུ་མཆི་
བར་བགྱི། །སེམས་ཅན་ཀུན་གྱི་དོན་གྱི་ཕྱིར། །
བདག་ནི་ཧེ་རུ་ཀར་གྱུར་ནས། །སེམས་ཅན་ཐམས་
ཅད་ཧེ་རུ་ཀའི། །གོ་འཕང་མཆོག་ལ་དགོད་པར་བགྱི།།
ལན་གསུམ། རྡོ་རྗེ་སེམས་དཔའི་བསྒོམ་བཟླས་ནི། རང་གི་སྤྱི་
བོ་པཾ་ལས་པདྨ་དང་། ཨ་ལས་ཟླ་བའི་གདན་གྱི་
སྟེང་དུ་ཧཱུྃ་ལས་རྡོ་རྗེ་དཀར་པོ་རྩེ་ལྔ་པ་ལྟེ་བ་ལ་ཧཱུྃ་གིས་
མཚན་པ། དེ་ལས་འོད་ཟེར་འཕྲོས། དོན་གཉིས་
བྱས་འདུས་ཡོངས་སུ་གྱུར་པ་ལས་རྡོ་རྗེ་སེམས་དཔའ་
དཀར་པོ་ཞལ་གཅིག་ཕྱག་གཉིས་རྡོ་རྗེ་དང་དྲིལ་བུ་འཛིན་
པ༔ རྡོ་རྗེ་སྐྱིལ་ཀྲུང་གིས་བཞུགས་པ། ཡུམ་རྡོ་
རྗེ་སྙེམས་མ་དཀར་མོ་ཞལ་གཅིག་ཕྱག་གཉིས་ཀྱི་གྲུག

ད

དང་ཕྱོད་པ་འཛིན་པས་འཁྲུད་པ། གཉིས་ཀ་འང་དར
དང་རིན་པོ་ཆེའི་རྒྱན་སྣ་ཚོགས་པས་སྤྲས་པ། གཉིས
ཀའི་སྤྱི་བོར་ཨོཾ། མགྲིན་པར་ཨཱཿ ཐུགས་ཀར་ཧཱུྃ།
ཐུགས་ཀའི་ཧཱུྃ་ལས་འོད་ཟེར་འཕྲོས་པས་རང་འདྲའི་ཡེ
ཤེས་པ་སྤྱན་དྲངས། །ཨོཾ་བཛྲ་རི་ཛི་ཧཱུྃ་ཧཱུྃ་ཕཊ། སྦ
ཟླ་ལྷབ་སྦྲུངས། སྟོང་པ་ཉིད་དུ་གྱུར། སྟོང་པའི་ངང
ལས་ཨཱཿ་ལས་ཕྱོད་པ་ཡངས་ལ་ཞིང་རྒྱ་ཆེ་བའི་ནང་དུ་ཀ་ལྷ
བདུད་རྩི་ལྷ་རྣམས་ཞབ་ལས་བྱུང་བའི་ཡེ་ཤེས་ཀྱི་བདུད
རྩི་རྒྱ་མཚོ་ཆེན་པོར་གྱུར། ཨོཾ་ཨཱཿ་ཧཱུྃ་ཧ་ཧོ་ཧྲཱིཿ ཞབ
གསུམ་གྲིམ་མཆོད་པ་བྱིན་རླབས་བྱ། རང་འདྲའི་ཡེ་ཤེས་པ་སྤྱན
དྲངས། ཨོཾ་བཛྲ་ས་ཏྭ་ཨརྒྷཾ་པྲ་ཏཱིཙྪ་ཧཱུྃ་སྭཱ་ཧཱ། ཞེས་པ་ནས།
ཤཔྟ་པྲ་ཏཱིཙྪ་ཧཱུྃ་སྭཱ་ཧཱ། ཛཿ་ཧཱུྃ་བཾ་ཧོཿ གཉིས་སུ་མེད
པར་གྱུར། སླར་ཡང་ཐུགས་ཀའི་ཧཱུྃ་ལས་འོད་ཟེར
འཕྲོས། དབང་གི་ལྷ་རྣམས་སྤྱན་དྲངས། ཨོཾ་པཉྩ
ཀུ་ལས་པ་རི་ཤུ་ར་ཨ་ཀྲྀན། ཤཔྟའི་བར་གྱི་མཆོད།
དེ་བཞིན་ག་ཤེགས་པ་ཐམས་ཅད་ཀྱིས་མངོན་པར་དབང
བསྐུར་དུ་གསོལ། ཞེས་གསོལ་བ་བཏབ་པས། དེ

༩

རྣམས་ཀྱིས་ཡེ་ཤེས་ཀྱི་བདུད་རྩིས་གང་བའི་ཐུཾ་པ་ཐོགས་
ནས༔ ཨོཾ་སརྦ་ཏ་ཐཱ་ག་ཏ་ཨ་བྷི་ཥེ་ཀ་ཏ་ས་མ་ཡ་ཤྲཱི་ཡེ་ཧཱུྃ།
ཞེས་དབང་བསྐུར། སྐུ་ཡེ་ཤེས་ཀྱི་བདུད་རྩིས་གང་།
མི་བསྐྱོད་པས་དབུ་བརྒྱན་ཅིང་། ཐུགས་ཀར་ཟླ་བའི་སྟེང་
དུ་ཧཱུྃ་གི་མཐར་ཡི་གེ་བརྒྱ་པའི་སྔགས་ཀྱིས་བསྐོར་བར་གྱུར།
ཨོཾ་བཛྲ་ས་ཏྭ་ཨཧཱུྃ་ནས། ཤབྟའི་བར་གྱིས་ཉེར་སྤྱོད་དང་། ཨོཾ་
བཛྲ་ས་ཏྭ་ཨོཾ་ཨཱཿཧཱུྃ་གིས་ནང་མཆོད་འབུལ། གཉིས་མེད་ཡེ་
ཤེས་འགྲོ་བའི་དཔལ། །མཆོག་ཏུ་མི་འགྱུར་བདེ་བ་ཆེས།།
སྡིག་ལྟུང་མ་ལུས་དྲུང་འབྱིན་པའི། །རྡོ་རྗེ་སེམས་མཆོག
ལ་ཕྱག་འཚལ། །མཆོད་ལ་བསྟོད་ནས། བདེ་སྟོང་ལྷན་ཅིག
སྐྱེས་པའི་ཡེ་ཤེས་ཀྱི། །གཟུང་རྣམས་ཞུང་ཁམས་སྐྱེ་
མཆེད་ལས་བྱུང་བའི། །རི་གླིང་རིན་ཆེན་གཏེར་བུམ་ཉི་
ཟླར་བཅས། །སྐྱབས་མགོན་ཐུགས་རྗེའི་གཏེར་ལ་དབུལ་
བར་བགྱི། །བདག་གི་ཆགས་སྡང་རྨོངས་གསུམ་སྐྱེ་
བའི་ཡུལ། །དགྲ་གཉེན་བར་གསུམ་ལུས་དང་ལོངས་
སྤྱོད་བཅས། །ཕངས་པ་མེད་པར་འབུལ་གྱི་ལེགས་
བཞེས་ནས། །དུས་གསུམ་རང་སར་གྲོལ་བར་བྱིན་གྱིས

༥

ཀློབས། །ཨོཾ་གུ་རུ་ར་ཏྣ་མཎྜལ་ཀཾ་ནི་རྻ་ཏ་ཡཱ་མི། །བཅོམ་
ལྡན་འདས་རྡོ་རྗེ་སེམས་དཔའ་བདག་གཞན་སེམས་ཅན་
ཐམས་ཅད་ཀྱི་སྡིག་སྒྲིབ་དང་དམ་ཚིག་ཉམས་ཆག་ཐམས་
ཅད་བྱང་ཞིང་དག་པར་མཛད་དུ་གསོལ། ཞེས་གསོལ་
བ་བཏབ་པས། ཐུགས་ཀའི་སྔགས་ཕྲེང་ཧཱུྃ་དང་བཅས་
པ་ལས་འོད་ཟེར་འཕྲོས། སེམས་ཅན་ཐམས་ཅད་ཀྱི་
སྡིག་སྒྲིབ་སྦྱངས། སངས་རྒྱས་སྲས་བཅས་ལ་མཉེས་
པའི་མཆོད་པ་ཕུལ། དེ་རྣམས་ཀྱི་སྐུ་གསུང་ཐུགས་
ཀྱི་ཡོན་ཏན་ཐམས་ཅད་འོད་ཀྱི་རྣམ་པར་བསྡུས་ནས་སྔགས་
ཕྲེང་ཧཱུྃ་དང་བཅས་པ་ལ་ཐིམ་པས། དེ་ལས་བདུད་རྩི་
རྒྱུན་དཀར་པོ་བབས་པ་ཡབ་ཡུམ་གྱི་སྦྱོར་མཚམས་ནས་
བབས། རང་གི་ཚངས་བུག་ནས་ཞུགས་ཏེ་ལུས་ཐམས་
ཅད་ཀྱི་ཡེ་ཤེས་ཀྱི་བདུད་རྩིའི་རྒྱུན་གྱིས་གང་། སྒོ་གསུམ་
གྱི་སྡིག་སྒྲིབ་ཐམས་ཅད་སངས་ཀྱིས་དག་པར་གྱུར།
ཨོཾ་བཛྲ་ཧེ་རུ་ཀ་ས་མ་ཡ། མ་ནུ་པཱ་ལ་ཡ། ཧེ་རུ་ཀ་
ཏྭེ་ནོ་པ་ཏིཥྛ་དྲྀ་ཌྷོ་མེ་བྷ་ཝ། སུ་ཏོ་ཥྱོ་མེ་བྷ་ཝ། སུ་
པོ་ཥྱོ་མེ་བྷ་ཝ། ཨ་ནུ་རཀྟོ་མེ་བྷ་ཝ། སརྦ་སིདྡྷི་མྨེ་པྲ

༨

ཡ་ཙྪ། སརྦ་ཀརྨ་སུ་ཙ་མེ། ཙིཏྟཾ་ཤྲཱི་ཡཾཿ ཀུ་རུ་ཧཱུྃ།
ཧ་ཧ་ཧ་ཧ་ཧོཿ བྷ་ག་ཝཱན། བཛྲ་ཧེ་རུ་ཀ་མཱ་མེ་མུཉྩ།
ཧེ་རུ་ཀ་བྷཱ་ཝ། མ་ཧཱ་ས་མ་ཡ་ས་ཏྭ་ཨཱཿ ཧཱུྃ་ཕཊ། ཉེར་
གཅིག་སོགས་བརྗོད། ཨོཾ་བཛྲ་ས་ཏྭ་ཨ་ཧཱུྃ་ཞེས་སོགས་དང་།
གཉིས་མེད་ཡེ་ཤེས་སོགས་ཀྱིས་བསྟོད། བདག་ནི་མི་ཤེས
རྨོངས་པ་ཡིས། །དམ་ཚིག་ལས་ནི་འགལ་ཞིང་ཉམས། །
བླ་མ་མགོན་པོས་སྐྱབས་མཛོད་ཅིག །གཙོ་བོ་རྡོ་རྗེ་འཛིན་
པ་སྟེ། །ཐུགས་རྗེ་ཆེན་པོའི་བདག་ཉིད་ཅན། །འགྲོ་
བའི་གཙོ་ལ་བདག་སྐྱབས་མཆི། །རྡོ་རྗེ་སེམས་དཔའི་
ཞལ་ནས་རིགས་ཀྱི་བུ་ཁྱོད་ཀྱི་སྡིག་སྒྲིབ་དང་དམ་ཚིག་ཉམས་
ཆགས་ཐམས་ཅད་བྱང་ཞིང་དག་གོ་ཞེས་གསུངས་ནས་རང་
ལ་ཐིམ་པས་རང་གི་སྒོ་གསུམ་དང་རྡོ་རྗེ་སེམས་དཔའི་སྐུ་
གསུང་ཐུགས་དབྱེར་མེད་པར་གྱུར། ། །
ཅེས་པ་འདི་ནི་ནུབ་ཕྱོགས་ཀྱི་གློ་ལྷུན་དུ་མཞེ་གནས་ལམ་རིམ་གྱི་གེགས་སེལ་བ་བཀོ་
འདོན་དང་། རིམ་གཉིས་བསྒོམ་པའི་སྔོན་འགྲོ་རྡོར་སེམས་ཀྱི་བསྙེན་བསྒྲུབ་ངག་
འདོན་ཞིག་དགོས་ཚེས་བསྐུལ་མ་བྱུང་བའི་རྐྱེན་བྱས། ཤུ་ནི་ཧྲཱི་ནའི་མིང་ཅན་གྱིས་
རྨོངས་ཚོད་བློ་བུར་དུ་བྲིས་པས་ན། བཟོད་པ་གསོལ། འཇམ་མགོན་རྒྱལ་

ཡོངས་ཐེག་པ་ཆེན་པོའི་སློབ་སྟོན་ཁང་ནས་ཕྱིར་བསྐྲུན་ཞུས་ཏེ་དོན་གཉེར་ཅན་
དག་ལ་འགྲེམས་སྤེལ་བགྱིས་པའོ།། །སརྦམངྒལཾ།། །།

༡

༄༅། །རྡོ་རྗེ་དམྱལ་བའི་གཉེན་པོ་ཚོགས་ཀྱི

འཁོར་ལོ་བདེ་ཆེན་དགའ་འཁྱིལ

ཞེས་བྱ་བ་བཞུགས་

སོ།།

༢

༄༅། །བཅོམ་ལྡན་འདས་ཀྱི་རྒྱུད་ལས་རྡོར་སེམས་བསྒོམ་བཟླས་ནི། ལམ་བསྐྱེད་རྫོགས་ཀྱི་རིམ་པ་བསྒོམ་པའི་སྔོན་འགྲོ་དང་། བར་དུ་ལམ་ཐབས་ཤེས་ཀྱི་སྒོམ་པ་ཡོངས་སུ་རྫོགས་པའི་གེགས་སེལ་བ་ཐོག་འདོན་གྱི་ཐབས་མཁས་སྨད་དུ་བྱུང་བར་གསུངས། དེ་ཡང་ཐོག་མར་རྒྱུད་སྡེ་ནང་དུ་སྒྲུབ་པའི་ཚེ་བླ་མ་དག་ལས་ལྷ་འདི་ཡི་སྐུ་གསུང་ཐུགས་ཡོན་ཏན་འཕྲིན་ལས་ཀྱི་རྗེས་གནང་དབང་བཞིའི་མོས་པ་དང་འབྲེལ་བའི་བྱིན་རླབས་ཅན་ཐོབ་པ་སྔོན་དུ་སོང་ནས་རྣལ་འབྱོར་པས་ལྷ་འདིའི་རྣལ་འབྱོར་རྒྱས་བསྡུས་ལ་གནས་ནས་རྡོ་རྗེ་དཀྱིལ་བའི་གཙོ་བོ་ཚོགས་ཀྱི་འཁོར་ལོའི་དགའ་སྟོན་ལ་ཧྲུག་རྒྱ་ཐུང་བ་ནི་སྐལ་བཟང་བདག་ནི་བདེ་བ་ཆེན་པོ་ལ་འཚེ་ཞིས་པ་ལྟར་རོ།། བླ་མེད་ལུགས་ཀྱི་རྡོར་སེམས་རྗེས་གནང་འདིའི་བརྒྱུད་པ་ནི་བདག་ལྷན་སྐྱེས་བརྒྱུད་ལས་བྱུང་བའི་མན་ངག་ཟབ་མོ་གཞན་ལ་མེད་པའི་ཕྱག་ཆོས་སུ་གྲུབ་དབང་ཧ་རུ་བདྲ་འི་གསུང་རྒྱུན་ལས་བྱུང་ཞིང་། དཀྱིལ་བར་ཕྱིན་རླབས་ཀྱི་བརྒྱུད་པའི་རྡོ་རྗེ་མ་ཡུལ་བར་འཛམས་ལེན་རང་གི་འགྲོན་བྱེད་རྒྱུ་ཡོད་པར་མོས་པའི་ལེགས་སྨོན་ཁྲ་ཏའི་ཚོགས་ཀྱིས་ཆོས་འདི་ལ་ནོར་བ་དང་། དེ་བྱེད་མཁན་ལ་བདུད་དུ་མ་འཛིན་ཅིག །དེ་ལྟར་ཕྱས་ན་ཕྱིད་དཀྱིལ་བར་གྱུར་ཏ་རེ།། གཙང་ཞིང་ཡིད་དུ་འོང་བའི་གཞལ་ཆང་བཟའ་བཅའི་རིགས་སོགས་ཀྱི་ཡོ་བྱད་ཅི་འབྱོར་བཤམས་ནས། ཚོགས་ཀྱི་ཞིང་དུ་བླ་མ་རྡོ་རྗེ་སེམས་དཔའི་དཀྱིལ་སྒོམ་པ་ནི། ཧཱུྃ༔ བདེ་སྟོང་གཉིས་

༣

སྐུ་མེད་པའི་རྣམ་རོལ་ལས། །བྱུང་བའི་རྡོ་རྗེ་སེམས

དཔའི་གཞལ་ཡས་ཁང་། །རྟེན་དང་བརྟེན་པའི

དཀྱིལ་འཁོར་ཡོངས་རྫོགས་མདུན། །ཀུན་བཟང

མཆོད་སྤྲིན་ནམ་མཁའི་ཁྱོན་ཀུན་ཁྱབ་གང་། །གཉིས

མེད་བདེ་བ་ཆེན་པོའི་མཁའ་དབྱིངས་ལ། །ངོ་མཚར

འགྲོ་རྣམས་ལྷ་དང་ལྷ་མོའི་འཕྲུལ། །ཞི་ཁྲོས་དབང

དྲག་སྤྲུལ་པའི་གར་མཁན་གྱི། །ཐབས་ཤེས་ཡོངས

སུ་རྫོགས་པའི་སྐུར་བཞེངས་གྱུར། །ཚོགས་རྫས་བྱིན

རླབས་བྱ་རྒྱུ་ལ་ནི། ཨོཾ་ཁཎྜ་རོ་ཧཱུྃ ས་བསངས། སྭ་བྷཱ་ཝས

སྦྱངས། སྟོང་པའི་ངང་ལས་ཨ་ལས་ཐོད་པ་ཡངས

ཤིང་རྒྱ་ཆེ་བའི་ནང་དུ་ཤ་ལྔ་བདུད་རྩི་ལྔ་རྣམས་ཞུ་བ་ལས

བྱུང་བའི་ཡེ་ཤེས་ཀྱི་བདུད་རྩིའི་རྒྱ་མཚོ་ཆེན་པོར་གྱུར།

ཨོཾ་ཨཱཿཧཱུྃ༔ཧ་ཧོ་ཧྲཱིཿ ལན་གསུམ། ཐམ་ལ་དབང

པོའི་ཡུལ་ལས་རབ་འདས་ཤིང་། །ཡོ་གེའི་དམ

ཚིག་དག་སྣང་བདེ་བ་ཆེ། །དངོས་གྲུབ་ཀུན་གྱི་གཞིར

གྱུར་བདུད་རྩིའི་མཆོག །རྟོག་མེད་བདེ་བ་ཆེན་པོའི

མཉེས་པར་མཛོད། །ཧཱུྃ༔ མཁའ་དབྱིངས་འཇའ

༨

ཚོན་རྡོ་རྗེ་སེམས་དཔའི་སྐུ། །བླ་མ་ཡི་དམ་མཁའ་...
འགྲོ་ཆོས་སྐྱོང་གི །ངོ་བོར་མ་རྟོགས་གཉིས་འཛིན་...
འཁྲུལ་སྣང་དག །དམ་རྫས་འདོད་ཡོན་སྣ་ལྔའི་ཚོགས་
མཆོད་ལ། །བླ་མ་རྡོ་རྗེ་སེམས་དཔའ་མཉེས་ཕྱིར་...
འབུལ། །ལྷན་སྐྱེས་བདེ་ཆེན་སྐྱེ་བར་བྱིན་གྱིས་རློབས།།
ཨོཾ་བཛྲ་ཧེ་རུ་ཀ་སམ་ཡ། མ་ནུ་པཱ་ལ་ཡ། ཧེ་རུ་ཀ།
ཏྭེ་ནོ་པ་ཏིཥྛ། དྲྀ་ཌྷོ་མེ་བྷ་ཝ། སུ་ཏོ་ཥྱོ་མེ་བྷ་ཝ།
སུ་པོ་ཥྱོ་མེ་བྷ་ཝ། ཨ་ནུ་ར་ཀྟོ་མེ་བྷ་ཝ། སརྦ་...
སིདྡྷིམྨེ་པྲ་ཡཙྪ། སརྦ་ཀརྨ་སུ་ཙ་མེ་ཙིཏྟཾ་ཤྲེ་ཡཾཿ
ཀུ་རུ་ཧཱུྂ། ཧ་ཧ་ཧ་ཧ་ཧོཿ བྷ་ག་ཝན། བཛྲ་ཧེ་རུ་ཀ་...
མ་མེ་མུཉྩ། ཧེ་རུ་ཀ་བྷ་ཝ། མ་ཧཱ་ས་མ་ཡ་ས་ཏྭ་...
ཨཱཿ ཧཱུྂ་ཕཊ། ཞེས་བརྗོད། ཧཱུྂཿ མཁའ་དབྱིངས་...
འཇའ་ཚོན་རྡོ་རྗེ་སེམས་དཔའི་སྐུ། །འདོད་ཡོན་བདེ་...
ལ་ཆགས་པའི་རྣམ་ཤེས་ལུས། །དཔལ་འབྱོར་དོན་...
མེད་བྱ་བའི་འཁྲུལ་སྣང་དག །དམ་རྫས་འདོད་ཡོན་...
སྣ་ལྔའི་ཚོགས་མཆོད་ལ། །བླ་མ་རྡོ་རྗེ་སེམས་དཔའ་...
མཉེས་ཕྱིར་འབུལ། །ཚེ་འདི་འི་སྣང་ཞེན་ལྡོག་པར་...

༥

བྱིན་གྱིས་རློབས། །ཨོཾ་བཛྲ་ཧེ་རུ་ཀ་ས་མ་ཡ་ ཞེས་སོགས་
བཟློད། ཧཱུྃ༔ མཁའ་དབྱིངས་འཇའ་ཚོན་རྡོ་རྗེ་སེམས་
པའི་སྐུ། །རྐྱུལ་མིན་ཡིད་བྱེད་རྣམ་རྟོག་ལས་ཅན་གྱི། །
སྒྲིབ་གཡོག་གཉིས་འཛིན་རིག་དོན་གྱི་འཁྲུལ་སྣང་དག །
དམ་རྫས་འདོད་ཡོན་སྣ་ལྔའི་ཚོགས་མཆོད་ལ། །བླ་
མ་རྡོ་རྗེ་སེམས་དཔའ་མཉེས་ཕྱིར་འབུལ། །ངེས་
འབྱུང་རྣམ་དག་སྐྱེ་བར་བྱིན་གྱིས་རློབས། །ཨོཾ་བཛྲ་ཧེ་རུ་
ཀ་ས་མ་ཡ་ ཞེས་སོགས་བཟློད། ཧཱུྃ༔ མཁའ་དབྱིངས་
འཇའ་ཚོན་རྡོ་རྗེ་སེམས་དཔའི་སྐུ། །རང་ཉིད་གཅེས་
འཛིན་སྡུག་བསྔལ་ཀུན་གྱི་སྒོ། །གཉིས་འཛིན་བདུད་
ཀྱི་འགོང་པོའི་འཁྲུལ་སྣང་དག །དམ་རྫས་འདོད་
ཡོན་སྣ་ལྔའི་ཚོགས་མཆོད་ལ། །བླ་མ་རྡོ་རྗེ་སེམས་
དཔའ་མཉེས་ཕྱིར་འབུལ། །རྣམ་དག་བྱང་སེམས་
སྐྱེ་བར་བྱིན་གྱིས་རློབས། །ཨོཾ་བཛྲ་ཧེ་རུ་ཀ་ས་མ་ཡ་
ཞེས་བཟློད། ཧཱུྃ༔ མཁའ་དབྱིངས་འཇའ་ཚོན་རྡོ་རྗེ་སེམས་
དཔའི་སྐུ། །རྟོག་པས་བར་བཞག་མིང་ཀྱང་བཏགས་
ཡོད་ལ། །གཉིས་འཛིན་དྲི་མ་ཅན་པའི་འཁྲུལ་སྣང་

༤

དག །དམ་རྫས་འདོད་ཡོན་སྣ་ལྔའི་ཚོགས་མཆོད་ལ།།
བླ་མ་རྡོ་རྗེ་སེམས་དཔའ་མཉེས་ཕྱིར་འབུལ། །ཕྱག་
རྒྱ་ཆེན་པོ་རྟོགས་པར་བྱིན་གྱིས་རློབས། །ཨོཾ་བཛྲ་ཧེ་རུ་
ཀ་ས་མ་ཡ་ ཞེས་སོགས་བརྗོད། ཧཱུྃ༔ མཁའ་དབྱིངས་
འཇའ་ཚོན་རྡོ་རྗེ་སེམས་དཔའི་སྐུ། །ཐ་མལ་སྣང་
ཞེན་ཀུན་རྟོག་ཕྲ་རགས་ཀྱི། །གཉིས་འཛིན་ནྲུང་ཁྲུ་
དྲག་པོའི་འཁྲུལ་སྣང་དག །དམ་རྫས་ཡེ་ཤེས་ལྔ་
ཡི་ཚོགས་མཆོད་ལ། །བླ་མ་རྡོ་རྗེ་སེམས་དཔའ་མཉེས་ཕྱིར་
ཧེས་དེ་དང་དབང་བཞི་ཐོབ་པར་བྱིན་གྱིས་རློབས། །ཨོཾ་
བཛྲ་ཧེ་རུ་ཀ་ས་མ་ཡ་ ཞེས་སོགས་བརྗོད། ཧཱུྃ༔ མཁའ་
དབྱིངས་འཇའ་ཚོན་རྡོ་རྗེ་སེམས་དཔའི་སྐུ། །ཉེས་
ལྟུང་དྲག་ཆར་དབང་མེད་བབས་པ་ལས། །རྡོ་རྗེ་དམྱལ་
བསྐྱོད་པའི་འཁྲུལ་སྣང་དག །དམ་རྫས་ཡེ་ཤེས་ལྔ་
ཡི་ཚོགས་མཆོད་ལ། །བླ་མ་རྡོ་རྗེ་སེམས་དཔའ་
མཉེས་ཕྱིར་འབུལ། །དག་པ་རབ་འབྱམས་འབབ་ཞིག་
འཆར་བར་ཤོག །ཨོཾ་བཛྲ་ཧེ་རུ་ཀ་ས་མ་ཡ་ ཞེས་སོགས་
བརྗོད། དེ་ནས་རྡོ་རྗེ་སློབ་དཔོན་ལ་ཚོགས་འབུལ་བ་ནི། རྡོ་རྗེ་

༥

འཛིན་པ་དགོངས་སུ་གསོལ། །དཔའ་བོ་དཔའ་མོ
ཚོགས་འཁོར་འདི། །གཟུང་དང་འཛིན་པའི་སྤྲོས་པ
བྲལ༔ ༔བདུད་རྩིའི་བདེ་ལ་རྟག་ཏུ་རོལ། །ཨ་ལ
ལ་ཧོ། །སློབ་དཔོན་གྱིས། ཨེ་མ་བདེ་ཆེན་ཡེ་ཤེས
ཀྱི༔ ༔ཚོགས་ཆེན་གཏུམ་མོ་འབར་བའི་དྲོད། །སྨྲ
བསམ་བརྗོད་འདས་དགའ་བདེ་ལ། །ཀུན་ཀྱང་ཨ་ཧོ
སུ་ཁ་ཆེ། །ཨ་ཧོ་མ་ཧཱ་སུ་ཁ་ཧོ། ཨོཾ་གུ་རུ་བཛྲ
ས་ཏྭ་ས་པ་རི་ཝཱ་ར་ཨ་མྲྀཾ་ནས་ཁ་ཧི་ཞེས་པར་གྱི་ཉེར་སྤྱོད་དང་།
གང་གི་མཚན་ཙམ་བརྗོད་པས་ཀྱང་། །ལས་ངན་སྒྲིབ
ལྟུང་མ་ལུས་པ། །སྐད་ཅིག་ཉིད་ལ་དྲུང་འབྱིན་པའི། །
རྡོ་རྗེ་སེམས་དཔའ་ལ་ཕྱག་འཚལ། །ཞེས་བསྟོད།
དེ་ནས་སྐང་བརྒྱུད་ཀྱིས་བསྟོད་པ་ནི། ཨོཾ་བཅོམ་ལྡན་དཔའ་བོའི
དབང་ཕྱུག་ལ་ཕྱག་འཚལ་ལ་ཧཱུྃ་ཧཱུྃ་ཕཊ། །ཨོཾ་བསྐལ་པ
ཆེན་པོའི་མེ་དང་མཚུངས་པའི་འོད་ཧཱུྃ་ཧཱུྃ་ཕཊ། །ཨོཾ
རལ་པའི་ཅོད་པན་མི་ཟད་པ་དང་ལྡན་ཧཱུྃ་ཧཱུྃ་ཕཊ། །ཨོཾ
མཆེ་བ་རྣམ་པར་གཙིགས་པ་འཇིགས་པའི་ཞལ་ཧཱུྃ་ཧཱུྃ་ཕཊ།།
ཨོཾ་སྟོང་ཕྲག་ཕྱག་ནི་འབར་བའི་འོད་ཟེར་ཅན་ཧཱུྃ་ཧཱུྃ་ཕཊ། །

༨

ཨོཾ་དྲ་ཤྲ་ཞགས་གདེངས་མ་དང་ དཔའ་བཏྣཾ་འཛིན་ཧཱུཾ་ཧཱུཾ་ཕཊ། །
ཨོཾ་སྟག་གི་པགས་པའི་ན་བཟའ་འཛིན་པ་ཅན་ཧཱུཾ་ཧཱུཾ་ཕཊ། །
ཨོཾ་སྐུ་ཆེན་དང་ཀ་བགེགས་མཐར་མཛད་ལ་འདུད་ཧཱུཾ་ཧཱུཾ་ཕཊ། །ཨོཾ་བཅོམ་ལྡན་འདས་མ་རྡོ་རྗེ་འཕགས་མོ་ལ་ཕྱག་འཚལ་ཧཱུཾ་ཧཱུཾ་ཕཊ། །ཨོཾ་འཕགས་མ་རིག་མའི་དབང་ཕྱུག་ཁམས་གསུམ་གྱིས་མི་ཐུབ་ཧཱུཾ་ཧཱུཾ་ཕཊ། །
ཨོཾ་འབྱུང་པོའི་འཇིགས་པ་ཐམས་ཅད་རྡོ་རྗེ་ཆེན་པོས་འཇོམས་ཧཱུཾ་ཧཱུཾ་ཕཊ། །ཨོཾ་རྡོ་རྗེ་གདན་བཞུགས་གཞན་གྱིས་མི་ཐུབ་དབང་བྱེད་ལྡན་ཧཱུཾ་ཧཱུཾ་ཕཊ། །ཨོཾ་གཏུམ་མོ་ཁྲོ་མོའི་གཟུགས་ཀྱིས་ཚེས་པ་སྐེམ་པར་མཛད་ཧཱུཾ་ཧཱུཾ་ཕཊ། །ཨོཾ་བདུད་རྣམས་སྐྲག་ཅིང་སྐེམ་པས་གཞན་གྱི་ཕྱོགས་ལས་རྒྱལ་ཧཱུཾ་ཧཱུཾ་ཕཊ། །ཨོཾ་རྨུག་བྱེད་རེངས་བྱེད་རྨོངས་བྱེད་ཀུན་ལས་རྣམ་པར་རྒྱལ་ཧཱུཾ་ཧཱུཾ་ཕཊ། །ཨོཾ་རྡོ་རྗེ་ཕག་མོ་སྦྱོར་བྱེད་འདོད་དབང་མ་ལ་འདུད་ཧཱུཾ་ཧཱུཾ་ཕཊ། །དེ་ནས་དངོས་གྲུབ་ཞུ་ཕྱིར་དཔྱིད་སྒྲ་གཏོང་། ཧཱུྃ། དེ་བཞིན་གཤེགས་པ་ཐམས་ཅད་དང་། །དཔའ་བོ་དང་ནི་རྣལ་འབྱོར་མ། །མཁའ་

འགྲོ་དང་ནི་མཁའ་འགྲོ་མ། །ཀུན་ལ་བདག་ནི་གསོལ་
བ་འདེབས། །བདེ་བ་ཆེ་ལ་དགྱེས་པའི་ཧེ་རུ་ཀ །
བས་རབ་མྱོས་མ་ལ་བསྟེན་བྱས་ནས། །ཆོ་ག
བཞིན་དུ་ལོངས་སྤྱོད་པ་ཡིས་ནི། །ལྷན་སྐྱེས་བདེ་བའི་
སྦྱོར་བ་ལ་ཞུགས་སོ། །ཨ་ལ་ལ། ལ་ལ་ཧོ།
ཨ་ཨི་ཨཱུཿ ཨ་ར་ལི་ཧོཿ དྲི་མེད་མཁའ་འགྲོའི་ཚོགས་
རྣམས་ཀྱིས། །བརྩེ་བས་གཟིགས་ལ་ལས་ཀུན་
མཛོད། །ཧཱུྃ། དེ་བཞིན་གཤེགས་པ་ཐམས་
ཅད་དང་། །དཔའ་བོ་དང་ནི་རྣལ་འབྱོར་མ། །
མཁའ་འགྲོ་དང་ནི་མཁའ་འགྲོ་མ། །ཀུན་ལ་བདག་ནི་
གསོལ་བ་འདེབས། །བདེ་བ་ཆེན་པོས་ཡིད་ནི་རབ་
བསྐྱོད་པས། །ལུས་ནི་ཀུན་ཏུ་གཡོ་བའི་གར་གྱིས་
ནི། །ཕྱག་རྒྱའི་པདྨར་རོལ་པའི་བདེ་བ་ཆེ། །རྣལ་
འབྱོར་མ་ཚོགས་རྣམས་ལ་མཆོད་པར་མཛད། །ཨ་
ལ་ལ། ལ་ལ་ཧོཿ ཨ་ཨི་ཨཱུཿ ཨ་ར་ལི་ཧོ།
དྲི་མེད་མཁའ་འགྲོའི་ཚོགས་རྣམས་ཀྱིས། །བརྩེ་
བས་གཟིགས་ལ་ལས་ཀུན་མཛོད། །ཧཱུྃ། དེ་

༡༠

བཞིན་གཤེགས་པ་ཐམས་ཅད་དང་། །དཔའ་བོ་དང་ནི་
རྣལ་འབྱོར་མ། །མཁའ་འགྲོ་དང་ནི་མཁའ་འགྲོ་མ། །
ཀུན་ལ་བདག་ནི་གསོལ་བ་འདེབས། །ཡིད་ཚོང་ཞི་
བའི་ཉམས་ཀྱི་གར་མཛད་མ། །རབ་དགྱེས་མགོན་པོ་
ཁྱོད་དང་མཁའ་འགྲོའི་ཚོགས། །བདག་གི་མདུན་དུ་
བཞུགས་ཏེ་བྱིན་རློབས་ལ། །ལྷན་སྐྱེས་བདེ་ཆེན་བདག་
ལ་སྩོལ་དུ་གསོལ། །ཨ་ལ་ལ། ལ་ལ་ཧོཿ ཨ་
ཨི་ཨཱཿ ཨ་ར་ལི་ཧོཿ དྲི་མེད་མཁའ་འགྲོའི་ཚོགས་
རྣམས་ཀྱིས། །བརྩེ་བས་གཟིགས་ལ་ལས་ཀུན་
མཛོད། །ཧཱུྃ། དེ་བཞིན་གཤེགས་པ་ཐམས་
ཅད་དང་། །དཔའ་བོ་དང་ནི་རྣལ་འབྱོར་མ། །མཁའ་
འགྲོ་དང་ནི་མཁའ་འགྲོ་མ། །ཀུན་ལ་བདག་ནི་གསོལ་
བ་འདེབས། །བདེ་ཆེན་ཐར་པའི་མཆོག་ཉིད་ལྡན་པ་
ཁྱོད༔ ༔བདེ་ཆེན་སྤངས་པའི་དཀའ་ཐུབ་དུ་མ་ཡིས། །
ཚེ་གཅིག་གྲོལ་བར་མི་བཞེད་བདེ་ཆེན་ཀྱང་། །ཆུ་སྐྱེས་
མཆོག་གི་དབུས་ན་གནས་པ་ཡིན། །ཨ་ལ་ལ།
ལ་ལ་ཧོཿ ཨ་ཨི་ཨཱཿ ཨ་ར་ལི་ཧོཿ དྲི་མེད་མཁའ

༄༅

འགྲོའི་ཚོགས་རྣམས་ཀྱིས། །བརྩེ་བས་གཟིགས་ལ
ལས་ཀུན་མཛོད། །ཧཱུྃ། དེ་བཞིན་གཤེགས་པ
ཐམས་ཅད་དང་། །དཔའ་བོ་དང་ནི་རྣལ་འབྱོར་མ། །
མཁའ་འགྲོ་དང་ནི་མཁའ་འགྲོ་མ། །ཀུན་ལ་བདག་ནི
གསོལ་བ་འདེབས། །འདམ་ཀྱི་དབུས་སུ་སྐྱེས་པའི
པདྨ་བཞིན། །ཆགས་པ་ལས་སྐྱེས་ཀྱང་ཆགས་པའི
སྐྱོན་མ་གོས། །རྣལ་འབྱོར་མ་མཆོག་པདྨའི་བདེ་བ
ཡིས། །སྲིད་པའི་མཆིང་བ་མྱུར་དུ་འགྲོལ་བར་མཛོད།།
ཨ་ལ་ལ། ལ་ལ་ཧོ༔ ཨ་ཨི་ཨཱ༔ ཨ་ར་ལི་ཧོ༔
དྲི་མེད་མཁའ་འགྲོའི་ཚོགས་རྣམས་ཀྱིས། །བརྩེ
བས་གཟིགས་ལ་ལས་ཀུན་མཛོད། །ཧཱུྃ། དེ
བཞིན་གཤེགས་པ་ཐམས་ཅད་དང་། །དཔའ་བོ་དང
ནི་རྣལ་འབྱོར་མ། །མཁའ་འགྲོ་དང་ནི་མཁའ་འགྲོ
མ། །ཀུན་ལ་བདག་ནི་གསོལ་བ་འདེབས། །སྦྲང
རྩིའི་འབྱུང་གནས་རྣམས་ཀྱི་སྦྲང་རྩིའི་བཅུད། །བུང
བའི་ཚོགས་ཀྱིས་ཀུན་ནས་འཐུང་བ་ལྟར། །མཚན་ཉིད
དྲུག་ལྡན་མཚོ་སྐྱེས་རྒྱས་པ་ཡིས། །བཅུད་བཅིངས

༡༢

པ་ཡི་རོ་ཡིས་ཚིམ་པར་མཛོད། །ཨ་ལ་ལ། ལ་ལ་
ཧོཿ ཨ་ཨི་ཨཱཿ ཨ་ར་ལི་ཧོཿ དྲི་མེད་མཁའ་འགྲོའི་
ཚོགས་རྣམས་ཀྱིས། །བརྩེ་བས་གཟིགས་ལ་ལས་
ཀུན་མཛོད། དེ་ནས་ཚོགས་ལྷག་འབུལ་བ་ནི། ཨོཾ་ཨཱཿཧཱུྃ་
ལན་གསུམ་བརྗོད། བདེ་སྟོང་དབྱེར་མེད་སྒྱུ་མའི་ཀ་པཱ་
ལར༔ ༔ཡེ་ཤེས་ལྷ་ཡི་བདུད་རྩིའི་ཚོགས་ལྷག་རྣམས། །
ཞིང་སྐྱོང་དྲེགས་པ་སྡེ་བརྒྱད་ཚོགས་ལ་འབུལ། །དམ་
ཚིག་སྲུང་བའི་ལས་བཞིའི་འཕྲིན་ལས་མཛོད།།
ཐུན་ཚོགས་དགེ་ལེགས་བྱེ་བའི་བསྐྲུན་པའི་སྐུ། །
མཐའ་ཡས་འགྲོ་བའི་རེ་བ་སྐོང་བའི་གསུང་། །འགྲོ་
བའི་བསམ་པ་ཇི་བཞིན་གཟིགས་པའི་ཐུགས། །རང་
སེམས་བླ་མར་མཇལ་བའི་བཀྲ་ཤིས་ཤོག །སྦྱང་
གཞིའི་འཆི་བར་བར་དོ་སྐྱེ་བ་གསུམ། །སྦྱོང་བྱེད་སྐུ་གསུམ་
ལམ་དུ་འཁྱེར་བའི་མཐུས། །རང་སེམས་གཅིག་
སེམས་ཕྲ་མོ་མཇལ་བ་ལས། །སྐུ་ཐུགས་ཟུང་
འཇུག་འཆར་བའི་བཀྲ་ཤིས་ཤོག །སྤྲོས་བྲལ་མཁའ་
དབྱིངས་སྟོང་པ་ཆེན་པོའི་ཡུམ། །སྣང་སྲིད་བདེ་བ་

༡༣

ཆེན་པོའི་ཡེ་ཤེས་ལ། །འབྱུང་བའི་ཡ་མཚན་འཁོར···

འདས་དངོས་པོ་ཀུན། །ཕད་སྟོང་ཆེན་པོར་སྡོམ······

མཛད་བཀྲ་ཤིས་ཤོག། །ཅེས་པ་འདི་ནི···

བོད་ལྗོངས་ལ་སོགས་པའི་འཛམ་གླིང་ཡུལ་གྲུ་མང་པོར་སྡོམ་པ་གསུམ་གྱི་བཅས་པ
དང་འགལ་འདུ་རམ་སོང་ན། འགྲོ་བ་མིའི་ཁྲལ་འདུ་མི་ཆུད་པའི་སྐབས་སྐྱེ་གསལ
ལས་ཀྱང་ཆེས་སྐྱིགས་མར་གྱུར་པས་ན། སྐལ་པ་དང་ལྡན་པའི་ཕྱོགས་ཀྱི···
རྣལ་འབྱོར་པ་རྣམས་ཀྱི་སྤྱི་གཙུག་འཛིམས་པ་ལ་ཤིན་ཏུ་དཔར་བའི་རྡོར་སེམས་ཀྱི···
ཉམས་ལེན་ལ་འཇུག་པ་ནི་བྱུང་འཇུག་བདེ་བ་ཆེན་པོའི་ཡེ་ཤེས་ཀྱི་དངོས་གྲུབ་ཐོབ···
པ་ལ་མེད་དུ་མི་རུང་བའི་གནས་སུ་མཐོང་སྟེ་ཕྱིར་བསོད་ནམས་ཀྱི་ཚོགས་ལྡབས་པོ
བསོགས་པ་དང་། དམ་ཚིག་ཉམས་ཆགས་སྐོང་བ། ལྷག་པར་རི་བོ···
དགེ་ལྡན་པའི་བླ་མ་དག་གིས་ནི་ཡིག་བརྒྱ་འབུམ་བཟླས་ནགས་རྟགས་ཀྱི་རྩ་ལྟུང···
ཡང་དག་པར་གསུངས་པ་སྐལ་འབྱོར་འདི་ས་མ་དག་པའི་སྒྲིབ་པ་མེད་པར་ཡིད···
ཆེས་པའི་གནས་སུ་གྲུངས་ཤིག། བཀྲིན་གསུམ་ལྡན་གྱི་རྩ་བའི་བླམ···
ངེས་པ་དོན་གྱི་ཧེ་རུ་ཀ་ཁྲི་ཆེན་རྡོ་རྗེ་འཆང་དམ་པའི་གསུང་དྲི་ཐབུ་ལུས་དཀྱིལ་གྱི······
བདག་འཇུག་ཉེ་ས་ལྷུང་དྲིམ་འབྱུང་བའི་ཆ་བརྒྱ་ནས་ཀྱང་། རིང་ནས་དྲིས་པའི
མཉེས་དང་བཅག་མེད་ཀྱིས། །ཉེས་ལྟུང་ཆར་བཞིན་བབས་པ་འདི་བསམ་ཆེ། །
དབང་མེད་རྡོ་རྗེའི་དམྱལ་བར་ལྷེར་གྱི་རྟོགས། །འོན་ཀྱང་རྒྱལ་བའི་ཐུགས་རྗེ···

༡༨

ཕྱིན་ཏུ་སྨྲར། །རྡོ་རྗེ་ཐེག་པའི་ཐབས་མཁས་མཆོག་ཏུ་ཟབ། །ཀུར་ཧྲི་ཆོག
རྨི་ལམ་བརྟེན་ནས་ཀྱང་། །ཉེས་ལྟུང་དྲུངས་ནས་འབྱིན་ འདི་ཨེ་མཧོ། །ཞེས
གསུངས་པ་སྟེར་རོ།། འདི་ནི་གནས་མཆོག་རྡོ་རྗེ་གདན་དུ་རང་གི་སློབ་མ
མདོ་སྔགས་ཟུང་འབྲེལ་གྱི་ལམ་ལ་གོ་བ་སྨྲ་དད་བྱུང་ཞིང་། ཐུབ་པའི་བསྟན་པ་ལ
ཡིད་ཆེས་ཀྱི་དད་པ་བརྟན་པོར་སྐྱེད་ནས་གསུམ་ལྷན་ཙར་སྐྱིག་གི་ཉམ་རོལ་བ་ཨེ་ཏར
ལེར་གི་སློབ་ཕྲུ་བ་བསྟན་དོན་ཡོད་ཀྱིས་ལྷག་བསམ་ཡིད་སྨོན་དང་འབྲེལ་ཡ་རྡོར་རོགས་དན
ཐུར་ཀུ་མ་ཤི་རྒྱ་དུ་འཛམ་གླིང་ཐེག་པ་ཆེན་པོའི་དགེ་འདུན་དང་མཉམ་དུ་མཆོད
སྤྲིན་སྨྲ་ལྷ་བརྒྱ ཚར་དང་། ཚོགས་ཀྱི་འཁོར་ལོ་སྟོང་ཚར་གྱི་འཇོག་སྒོར
ཚིག་ཁྲི་བརྒྱད་སྟོང་བཅས་འབུལ་པར་དགོས་ཀྱི་རྐྱེན་ལས། ཕྱི་ལོ་ ༡༩༨༣
ཟླ་ ༢ ཚེས་ ༣ བོད་རྒྱལ་ལོ་ ༢༡༠༨ ཟླ་ ༠༢ ཚེས་ ༡༠
མཁའ་འགྲོ་འདུ་བའི་དུས་ཆེན་ཉིན་སྒྲོགས་བཅུ་འི་དགེ་འདུན་རྣམས་ཐུགས་མཐུན
ཁྲིམས་གཙང་རྟོགས་ལམ་བསླབ་པ་གསུམ་གྱི་ཉམས་ལེན་མཐར་ཕྱིན་ཏེ་སེམས
ཅན་གྱི་དོན་རྒྱ་ཆེན་པོ་མཛད་པར་གྱུར་པའི་སྨོན་ཚིག་དང་བཅས་རང་སྣང་གང་དྲན་ཆེ་གེས
སུ་སྨྲ་བར་འདོད་པའི་རིག་ཁྱབ་ཅན་གྱི་རྡོ་རྗེ་སེམས་དཔའི་ཞབས་ལ་འཁོར་བ་ཀུན་ཏུའི་དགེ
སློང་མུ་ནི་ཧཾ་ནའི་མིང་ཅན་གྱིས་སུག་བྲིས་བགྱིས་པའོ།། །།

༄ གསེར་གྱིས་གཞི་ཕྲུག་ས་སྤོམ་རི་བོང་ནས། །བཟང་གི་དོགས
ནས་སྣང་སྲིད་དཔྲ་དུ་ཤར་ཀས། །ཐུབ་མཆོག་ཡམ་དང་དབང་གི་བརྒྱུད་མཐྱེན། །

༡༥

ནམ་མཁའི་བརྡོ་འི་ཡོ་གི་ར་འཁྲུལ་ལ་མཆིར། ། ཞེས་ཀྱང་གསུངས་སོ།། ||

༢ ཚོགས་ཚོས་འདི་ནི་བླ་མེད་ཀྱི་ཡི་དམ་གཞན་ཡང་རུང་སྟེ་ཚོགས་བཏང་ན་སྒྲིགས་

པར་སེམས་ཏེ། དབེར་ན་བླ་མེད་ཀྱི་སྒྲོལ་མར་སྒྲུར་ན་རང་སྒྲོལ་མའི་རྣལ་འབྱོར་

ལ་གནས་ནས་ཚོགས་ཀྱི་ཞིང་དུ་བླ་མ་སྒྲོལ་མའི་དཀྱིལ་འཁོར་སྒོམས་པའི་སྐབས་ །

སྒྲུབ་པའི་འཕགས་མ་སྒྲོལ་མའི་གཞལ་ཡས་ཁང་། ། ཞེས་དང་། མཁའ་

དབྱིངས་འཇའ་འོད་ཚོན་འཕགས་མ་སྒྲོལ་མའི་སྐུ། ། ཞེས་དང་། སྒྲོལ་མ་

ཉེར་གཅིག་ལས་བདུད་རྩི་འོད་ཟེར་དང་བཅས་རང་ལ་ཐིམ་པའི་དམིགས་རྣམ་སྐྱོང་

བཞིན་པར་ཐམས་ལ་སྣང་ཞེན་གྱི་འཕྲས་བུ་ཉེས་ལྟུང་ཐམས་ཅད་དག་པར་བསམ་སྟེ་

སྒྲོལ་མའི་སྔགས་ཉེར་གཅིག་བགྲང་ངོ།། གསང་བདེ་འཇིགས་

གསུམ་སོགས་ལ་འང་དེ་བཞིན་དུ་རང་རང་གི་བདག་བསྐྱེད་རྫོགས་བསྡུས་ལ་གནས་

ནས་མཆོད་པ་ བྱིན་རླབས་ཀྱི་འགྲོ་ལྟར་དང་། ཡང་ན་རང་རང་གི་འགྲོ་

ལྟར་བྱའོ།། ལྟར་བཞིན་དམིགས་རྣམས་སྐྱོང་བའམ་ཏིང་ངེ་འཛིན་གྱི་

དབང་བཞི་ལེན་པའི་དམིགས་པ་ལྟར་བྱས་ཏེ་སྙིང་པོ་དང་། ཉེ་སྙིང་ཉེར་

ཅིག་སོགས་རྒྱས་བསྡུས་ཅི་རིགས་བྱའོ།། ||

༢ དཔེ་ཆ་ལྷ་བརྒྱ་ཐམ་པ་འཇམ་མགྲིན་ཐེག་པ་ཆེན་པོའི་དགེ་འདུན་གྱི་ཚོགས་

འདོན་ཆེད་ཚེས་ཚོགས་ལུགས་ཡོན་སྒྲུར་ཏེ་ཞེས་རིགས་ཐར་ཁང་དུ་ཕྱར་འདེབས་ཆེད་

ཡི་གེ་པའི་ངོ་མིན་བྱང་ཆུབ་ཚོས་གླིང་གི་སློབ་གཉེར་བ་དགེ་ཚུལ་ནོར་བུ་ལམ

༢༨

བཟང་པོ། །བཀྲ་ཤིས་སན་མདྲ་ལཾ། །

དགེའོ། བཀྲ་ཤིས། རྗེ་རྒྱུད་བླ་མ་རྣམས་ཀྱི་བྱིན---

རླབས་དང་། །ཡི་དམ་རྡོ་རྗེ་སེམས་དཔའི་དངོས་གྲུབ་ཆེ། །

གནས་གསུམ་མཁའ་འགྲོ་ཚོགས་སྐྱོང་འཕྲིན་ལས་ཀྱིས། །འགྲོ་

ཀུན་གཙན་བདེས་ཚིམ་པས་བཀྲ་ཤིས་ཤོག། །

Appendix 4

Translation and Explanation of the One Hundred Syllable Mantra

Translation and Explanation of the One Hundred Syllable Mantra

OM VAJRA HERUKA SAMAYAM ANUPALAYA. HERUKA TENOPATISHTHA. DRIDHO ME BHAVA, SUTOSHYO ME BHAVA, SUPOSHYO ME BHAVA, ANURAKTO ME BHAVA. SARVA SIDDHIM ME PRAYACCHA. SARVA KARMA SUCHA ME CHITTAM SHREYAH KURU HUM! HA HA HA HA HOH! BHAGAVAN VAJRA HERUKA MA ME MUNCHA. HERUKA BHAVA MAHA SAMAYA SATTVA AH HUM PHAT!

OM is the seed syllable that symbolizes the divine vajra body, that is, the holy body of an enlightened being. The vajra body is union-oneness with divine vajra speech and mind. At present, your body, speech, and mind function separately, but when you attain the enlightened state of Heruka Vajrasattva your divine body, speech, and mind will function simultaneously.

VAJRA HERUKA. The pure energy of the indestructible divine wisdom thought of the greatest, blissful, innermost heart, which encompasses all phenomena.

SAMAYAM. When during an initiation you give your sacred word of honor to keep your vows and pledges purely, a subtle energy is generated within your mind and inner nervous system. This energy automatically releases you from negativity. This is what samaya means. It is the exact opposite of the half-hearted promises people usually make; promises that are so easily broken. Where your samaya is involved, you should not rationalize, even for the sake of your life.

ANUPALAYA. The power of divine loving kindness, which can bring you to eternal happiness.

HERUKA TENOPATISHTHA. Magnificent Heruka, be close within my heart.

DRIDHO. Indestructible, eternal, never-changing.

ME BHAVA. Grant me the divine, indestructible wisdom of the realization of the absolute true nature of myself and all other universal phenomena.

SUTOSHYO ME BHAVA. Vajrasattva, through being close to me, grant me the greatest, joyful divine wisdom, which brings great bliss.

SUPOSHYO ME BHAVA. May this blissful energy develop perfectly within my heart.

ANURAKTO ME BHAVA. May I be influenced by the divine attachment reflection of compassionate wisdom, which is utterly beyond duality.

SARVA SIDDHIM ME PRAYACCHA. Grant me completely all magnificent realizations.

SARVA KARMA SUCHA ME. Grant me all divine wisdom actions of Vajrasattva.

CHITTAM SHREYAH KURU. May your magnificent divine wisdom function in my heart.

HUM. The seed-syllable that symbolizes the nature of the divine vajra heart, the greatest divine blissful wisdom.

HA HA HA HA HOH. These five syllables symbolize the five wisdoms of the five dhyani buddhas.

BHAGAVAN. The enlightened one.

VAJRA HERUKA. The greatest, indestructible blissful wisdom.

MA ME MUNCHA. Do not abandon me.

HERUKA BHAVA. Be indestructibly held in my heart, by my keeping indestructible samaya, just as you hold the indestructible vajra.

MAHA. Greatest.

SAMAYA. As above.

SATTVA. The divine wisdom thought.

AH. The seed-syllable symbolizing divine vajra speech.

HUM. As above.

PHAT! Destroy all negative distractions!

Appendix 5

Blessing the Shi-dak Torma

OM VAJRA AMRITA KUNDALI HANA HANA HUM PHAT!
OM SVABHAVA SHUDDHA SARVA DHARMA SVABHAVA SHUDDHO HAM!

Tong-pa nyid-du gyur.
Tong-päi ngang-lä DRUNG-lä rin-po-che nö-yang shing-gya che-wä nang-du OM-ö du-zhu wa-lä jung-wä tor-ma zag-pa me-pä ye-she kyi dü-tsi gya-tso chen-por gyur

OM AH HUM *(say three times)*
NAMA SARVA TATHAGATA AVALOKITE OM SAMBARA SAMBARA HUM
(say three times)

Chom-dän de-zhin shek-pa gyäl-wa rin-chen mang-la chak tsäl-lo
De-zhin shek-pa zug-tse dam-pa-la chak tsäl-lo
De-zhin shek-pa ku-jam lä-la chak tsäl-lo
De-zhin shek-pa jig-pa tham-chä dang-dräl wa-la chak tsäl-lo

Pün-tsok dö-yön nga-dän pa
Dü-tsi gya-tso tor-ma di
Sa-yi lha-mo te-ma sok
Tong-sum shi-dak tham-chä dang
Tse-ring chä-nga ten-kyong gi
Gang-chen nä-pa tham-chä dang
Kye-par yu-jor de-nyi kyi
Lha-lü shi-dak nam-la bül
Zhe-nä dak-chak yön-chö nam
Lä-dang ja-wa chi-chi kyang
Kor-long tra-dok ma-tse pa

BLESSING THE SHI-DAK TORMA[38]

OM BENDZA AMRITA KUNDALI HANA HANA HUM PHAT!
OM SVABHAVA SHUDDHA SARVA DHARMA SVABHAVA SHUDDHO HAM!

All becomes empty.
From within emptiness, from DRUNG, comes a broad, vast jewelled vessel, inside of which, from OM melting into light, there arises a torma of a great ocean of undefiled nectar of wisdom.

OM AH HUM *(say three times)*
NAMA SARVA TATHAGATA AVALOKITE OM SAMBARA SAMBARA HUM *(say three times)*

I prostrate to the bhagawan, the tathagata Many Jewelled One (Bahuratna)
I prostrate to the tathagata Supreme Beautiful Form (Varasurupa)
I prostrate to the tathagata Infinite-Bodied One (Paryantakaya)
I prostrate to the tathagata Free From All Fear (Sarvabhayashri)

This torma, an ocean of nectar
Endowed with the five perfect sensual objects,
I offer to Tema, goddess of the earth,
And all land owners of the three thousand worlds;
To the five sister goddesses of long life,
And all protectors of stability who reside in Tibet.
And especially to the devas, nagas,
And land owners dwelling in this very region.
Having accepted, I request you to gather, as we wish,
All harmonious conditions for whatever actions
We and the sponsors perform

Tün-kyen yi-shin drub-par tzö
Dak-gi sam-pä tob-dang ni
De-zhin shek-pä jin-tob dang
Chö-kyi ying-gi tob-nam kyi
Dön-nam gang-dak sam-pa yi
De-dak tham-chä chi-rik pa
Tok-pa me-par jung-gyur chik

Without showing anger or jealousy.
By the power of my thoughts,
By the power of the blessings of the tathagatas,
And by the power of the sphere of reality,
May any purpose we desire,
All whatsoever, be realized without obstruction!

NOTES

1. Wisdom Archive numbers 000154, –166, –392, and –596.
2. See *Liberation in the Palm of Your Hand,* pp. 216–23 (the four opponent powers) and pp. 430–70 (karma).
3. This is in 1974, when there were only two, very basic toilets: Sam and Sara!
4. See Lama Yeshe's *Bliss of Inner Fire,* which contains his teachings on tum-mo from the Six Yogas of Naropa.
5. In 1981–82 Lama Yeshe prepared his first batch of chu-len pills according to traditional procedures, using extremely valuable natural ingredients detailed in a booklet published by Wisdom at the time. The pills were then blessed through the recitation of one million Heruka Vajrasattva mantras. In the summer of 1982, using these pills under the leadership of the late great yogi Geshe Jampa Wangdu, fifty Dharma students from all over the world made successful retreats at Tushita Retreat Centre, Dharamsala, India, showing that this practice is no longer for Tibetans alone. These fasting retreats are still conducted at some FPMT centers, using pills made by the Tibetan Medical and Astrological Institute, Dharamsala.
6. See *Introduction to Tantra,* pp. 129 ff.
7. See appendix 4 for a translation and explanation of this mantra.
8. See Lama Zopa Rinpoche's *Direct & Unmistaken Method* for complete instructions on taking precepts.
9. Some people also place a fourth torma in the offering bowl that represents the food offering, as shown in the altar drawing. Otherwise, this bowl would contain some other food or water. Whatever it contains should be offered daily. Lama Zopa Rinpoche emphasizes that other food can replace traditional tormas, as mentioned by Lama Yeshe. There are many variations in these ritual matters, and you

should consult your lama to see what you should do.

10. A short way of blessing the torma is as follows: First recite HA HO HRI three times with your hands in the correct mudra, left above the right, open, facing forward, thumbs pointing right. With this recitation, all faults of color, smell, taste, and potentiality are purified, and the torma becomes blissful nectar. Then recite OM AH HUM three times. The nectar increases vastly and is blessed. Visualize that it becomes inexhaustible. After that, make the outer offering: OM VAJRASATTVA ARGHAM...SHABTA PRATICCHA HUM SVAHA. Finally, recite the praise *Nyi-me ye-she...* from the sadhana, substituting *...ch'ak-s'äl-tö* (homage and praise) for *...la-ch'ak-ts'äl* in the last line. For a longer blessing ritual, you can perform the inner offering from, for example, the Vajrayogini sadhana, or the blessing of the Heruka Vajrasattva tsog as explained in part 4 of this book.

11. Geshe Tsulga, of Sera-je Monastic University (and resident teacher at the FPMT's American east coast centers), explains that you can offer this torma every day, visualizing that you are offering a "fresh" bit of it each time; or, you can place a biscuit or other food offering beside this torma and offer that as the principal torma each day. The best time to offer this torma is during the last session of the day. After the mantra recitation, before the offering and praise, bless the torma as above; then visualize that letters HUM on the tongues of Heruka Vajrasattva and Yum Nyem-ma Kar-mo transform into hollow tubes of rainbow light the width of a wheat grain in diameter. With recitation of the mantra OM VAJRASATTVA SAPARIVARA IDAM BALINTA KAKA KAHI KAHI, these radiate out to the torma and extract its essence, great bliss. Then return to the sadhana.

12. The special protector is Four-Armed Mahakala. Ideally you should offer this torma three times: once at the beginning of retreat, next around the middle, and finally, when your retreat has finished. The Mahakala *kang-sö* (fulfillment and restoration) ritual can be performed when you make this offering.

13. Lama Zopa Rinpoche says that this third torma offering can be done just once, at the beginning of the retreat. However, it can also be done every day, or three times during the retreat, along with the Mahakala kang-sö, as above. See appendix 5 for a ritual for blessing the shi-dak torma.

14. See *Liberation in the Palm of Your Hand*, p. 146, for more benefits of offering water.

15. The same applies to the Heruka Vajrasattva tsok puja. Geshe Tsulga says that in retreat, it would be good to do the Heruka Vajrasattva tsok daily, as long as it doesn't prevent you from reaching your goal of one hundred thousand mantras. You should definitely do it on the tenth and the twenty-fifth of each Tibetan month, the usual tsok days.

16. Geshe Tsulga explains that for a perfect accumulation and to receive the blessings of Heruka Vajrasattva swiftly, powerfully, and continually, you should recite the *ye-she pä-nga*. After you have finished one hundred thousand Vajrasattva mantras, recite another ten thousand (i.e., ten percent of the total), substituting the syllables HA ANDZE SVAHA for the PHAT at the end of the usual mantra. Thus, it now finishes ...SAMAYA SATTVA AH HUM HA ANDZE SVAHA. The Dorje Khadro fire puja can be done after this.

17. Geshe Tsulga says that you need to count one hundred thousand mantras and do a fire puja to be qualified to do certain activities, such as those mentioned in a manual compiled by the Tibetan lama Ngul-chu Dharmabhadra. Self-initiation is one example of these. Of course, you can do a fire puja no matter how many mantras you have counted, but if it's under one hundred thousand, you won't be qualified to do the special activities. Each deity has its own collection of activities (*lä-tsok*).

18. Tib: *tsa-me-nga*; literally, "five no choice." It means you have no choice but to be reborn in hell when the life in which you created that action has finished.

19. See pp. 154–55, where Lama explains why he sometimes *doesn't* do this.

20. The principal object of refuge can also be Vajradhara, as Lama explains in the main commentary.

21. See note 18, above. While in common terms these five are "inexpiable" sins, the powerful methods of tantra do allow you to purify them.

22. See also "The meditation seat," pp. 74 ff., and pp. 152–53, where Lama explains how to make a portable meditation seat.

23. Lama Yeshe organized the first Enlightened Experience Celebration (EEC), a large international gathering of his Western students, at Bodhgaya, India, in 1982. This six-month series of teachings, initiations, and retreats was attended by more than two hundred students, almost one hundred of whom were monks and nuns. Since Lama passed away, Lama Zopa Rinpoche has organized two more EECs, with the fourth scheduled for 1995–96.

24. See, for example, Lama Yeshe, Cittamani Tara commentary (transcript), Kopan, January/February, 1979, lectures 5–7.

25. See *Introduction to Tantra,* p. 111.

26. Sadly, this was indeed Lama's last talk at Vajrapani Institute. Despite his assurances, a few months later, in Nepal, his health began to deteriorate rapidly, and he passed away in Los Angeles on March 1, 1984. A few days later, Lama was cremated at Vajrapani, where a beautiful stupa has been erected in his memory.

27. The translation of the sadhana presented here combines Lama Yeshe's original translation, which was interspersed with commentary, and Martin Willson's version, found in the transcript *Heruka Vajrasattva: Sadhana and Ritual Feast* (Boston: Wisdom Publications, 1984), a literal translation of Lama's Tibetan text.

28. This interpretive translation was made by Jon Landaw, working together with Lama Yeshe, Lama Zopa Rinpoche, and Ven. Konchog Yeshe. Some suggested corrections were made later by Thubten Chödak and Piero Cerri. Martin Willson's literal translation of the introduction (see note 27) follows:

> In the tantras of the Lord, it is taught that meditation and mantra recitation of Vajrasattva is an excellent skillful means as a preliminary to practicing the developing and completing stages of the path, and for producing profit and eliminating hindrances to perfect practice of method and wisdom at the intermediate stages of the path.
>
> Initially, to make your continuum a fit vessel, you should receive from the gurus the permission (*je-nang*) of the body, speech, mind, qualities, and activities of this deity, having blessing connected with conviction towards the four empowerments. The practitioner who has done this and is abiding in the long or short yoga of this deity [i.e., you must have generated yourself as the deity, either by the full sadhana or by a shorter method such as that given in the section

"Preliminaries" (see note 29, below)] has the chance to begin *The Banquet [of Great Bliss]: The Ritual Feast that Counters the Vajra Hells*; as has been said: "Fortunate am I in great bliss."

The transmission of this permission of Vajrasattva in the highest yoga tantra tradition is that it comes from the speech of the lord of the *siddhas* Dharmavajra as a special teaching not found except in the profound oral instructions of the ear[-whispered] lineage of Gadän. Until now the warmth of the transmission of the blessings is undiminished; the practice is there for oneself to do, now it has reached [one]. Do not hold through a flock of magpie-like, deluded wrong prayers that this teaching is erroneous and its practitioners are devils (*mara*). If you do, you will surely go to hell.

29. This last paragraph is not in the text but is from an explanation of tsok given to Jon Landaw by Lama Yeshe while they were working on the translation. We felt it was helpful to include it here.

30. *Bala* and *madana*: Sanskrit terms for the sacramental offerings of meat and alcohol respectively. Although meat and alcohol might be how these substances appear to ordinary perception, they should not be thought of as such, but should instead be seen in their true nature of simultaneously born bliss and void and always referred to as "bala" and "madana."

31. The Heruka Vajrasattva sadhana given in appendix 1 is an elaborate meditation for generating yourself as the deity. The following abbreviated method was suggested by Lama Zopa Rinpoche:

    a) Take refuge and generate bodhicitta

    b) Meditate on the four immeasurables

    c) Do the special generation of bodhicitta, for example: "In particular, for the sake of all mother sentient beings, quickly, quickly I must somehow obtain the precious state of complete and perfect buddhahood. Therefore, I shall practice the yoga of the profound path of Guru Vajrasattva."

    d) Recite the *Hundreds of Deities From the Land of Joy (Ga-dän lha-gyä-ma),* followed by the *Mik-tse-ma.*

    e) Do a glance meditation on the lam-rim, for example, the *Foundation of All Good Qualities (Yön ten zhir gyur ma)* by Lama Tsong Khapa or the lam-rim prayer from the *Guru Puja.*

f) Then, the Lama Tsong Khapa visualized in front of you absorbs into your heart, and you become one with him. If you have received an empowerment of highest yoga tantra, experience non-dual bliss and void. Then, that which you label "I" manifests as Vajrasattva.

32. Lama Zopa Rinpoche suggests (letter to students, March 27, 1984) that as you offer the tsok with each verse, think that it generates great bliss in the mind of Guru Vajrasattva, who is the embodiment of all gurus, Buddha, Dharma, and Sangha.

33. As you recite the mantra, you can practice the män-de, yän-de, and phung-de purifications as explained in the commentary. Lama Zopa adds:

    Visualize strong nectar and light rays flowing from Guru Vajrasattva, completely purifying all sentient beings' obscurations and negative karma, including any particular problem being experienced by some being for whom you'd like to pray. All realizations of the entire path, especially those mentioned in the immediately preceding verse, are generated in your own and all other sentient beings' minds.

34. Martin Willson made his translation from a Tibetan text printed at the She-rig Par-khang (from which the Tibetan text in appendix 3 was copied). It seems that Lama Yeshe later added a little material to the version that Jon Landaw translated. The end matter from Martin Willson's translation is as follows:

    a) Conclusion. If in Tibet and many other countries of the world [the times] are not totally incompatible with the rules of the three vowed disciplines, [still] they are more degenerate by far even than the degenerations in cases of destinies not included in the human. Therefore, fortunate mantric practitioners should see that undertaking the practice of Vajrasattva, who is very brave in overcoming their sins and offences, is a basis indispensable for attaining the realization of the wisdom-knowledge of the great bliss of unification. And since, in general, it powerfully gathers the accumulation of merits and makes good damaged and broken pledges, and since it has especially been taught by Geluk lamas that reciting one hundred thousand one hundred syllable mantras will purify even tantric downfalls, you should take it as something you can depend on that this yoga annihilates impure evil.

As my root guru endowed with the three kindnesses, the Heruka of definitive meaning, Trijang Dorje Chang, has said in his holy teaching, *Self-entry to the Body Mandala of Ganta[pada Shri Chakrasamvara]: A Stream of Water Washing Off the Dirt of Misdeeds and Offences*:

When we think that through long-familiar delusion
And recklessness, faults and offences pour down like rain,
We fear being helplessly driven to vajra hell.
Yet most swift is the Conqueror's compassion—
Relying on a short but most profound rite,
The skilled in Vajrayana can
Uproot offences and misdeeds—how marvellous!

b) Colophon. At Vajrasana (Bodhgaya), a disciple of mine with remarkable undersanding of the path uniting sutra and tantra, who, having found firm, confident faith in the teachings of the Sage (Shakyamuni Buddha), manifests in saffron, possessing the three [vowed disciplines], the Italian *ge-long* Thubten Dönyö, with the wish of special intention, offered under the Bodhgaya bodhi tree in the company of an international Mahayana sangha [members of the International Mahayana Institute] a hundred fivefold offering-clouds, a thousand ritual feasts, and 18,000 rupees for general purposes.

Because of this need, on the third day of February 1982, the tenth day of the twelfth month of the Tibetan year 2108, the day of the great gathering of dakinis, praying that the Sangha of the ten directions may be harmonious and pure in morality, reach the end of the practice of the three trainings of the direct path, and perform extensive benefit for sentient beings, and wishing to say in words what I recall seeing, I, a prattling practitioner of Vajrasattva, the Buddhist monk called Muni Jñana, have written this by hand.

This too is said:

From fear that the golden ground be shattered
By a rabbit's horn of tantric vows,
All existence rises as one's foe.
Strange, if minds not ripened by empowerment

And the common path transformed by magic

Into yogins, like sky-lotuses!

c) Adaptation for use with other deities. This ritual feast may also be adapted for offering a ritual feast to other deities of highest yoga tantra. To adapt it to the highest yoga tantra aspect of Tara, for example, [do the following]: abiding in the yoga of Tara (i.e., visualizing yourself as Tara), visualize as the field for the accumulation [of merit] the mandala of Guru Tara. At this point (first verse of the visualization of the mandala of Vajrasattva), say, "*Jung-wäi pak-ma Dröl-mäi zhäl-yä-kang* (Appears before me the palace of Arya Tara....)" In the offering verses (verses 1 through 7) say "*Ka-ying Ja-tsön pak-ma Dröl-mäi ku* (Rainbow in space that is Arya Tara's body!" [and adapt the fifth line similarly].

[After each verse,] keeping the visualization that from the twenty-one Taras nectar and light rays dissolve into you, think that all offences and misdeeds, the results of clinging to ordinary appearance, are purified, while you recite Tara's mantra twenty-one times.

Similarly for Guhyasamaja, Heruka, Yamantaka, or others, perform the corresponding long or short self-generation, and abiding in this, consecrate the offerings by either the general procedure or (that deity's) special procedure. Keeping the above visualization, or doing a visualization like that for taking the four empowerments in concentration, recite the heart and near-heart mantras twenty-one times or more, long or short as is practicable.

35. Thub(ten) Yeshe in Sanskrit: Muni(shasana) Jñana.

36. See above for a more literal translation. Jon Landaw worked on this version with Lama Yeshe and says that taking the liberty of putting it into English verse necessitated a little license with the vocabulary. He also mentions that "the hardest point to render was in stanza one. The phrase 'rabbit's horn of tantric ordination' means that the person, who is so fearful of breaking his samaya that he sees everything as his enemy, never really received the empowerment in the first place. Thus, for him the initiation was like a rabbit's horn.... I tried to re-emphasize [this point] in line three of the second stanza."

37. At the very end of the end matter, the Tibetan text has a final verse of auspiciousness that does not appear to have been translated by either Jon Landaw or Martin Willson. In phonetics, this reads:

Tsa-gyü la-ma nam-kyi jin-lab dang
Yi-dam Dor-je Sem-päi ngö-drub che
Nä-sum kha-dro chö-kyong trin-lä kyi
Dro-kün tän-de tsim-pä tra-shi-shog

An edited version of a translation of this verse provided by Thubten Chödak and Piero Cerri reads:

Through the blessings of all the root and lineage lamas,
The great accomplishments of the mind-bound deity Vajrasattva, and
The divine actions of the dakinis and protectors of the three places,
May auspiciousness allow all beings to be satisfied by ultimate peace!

38. Thanks to David Molk for providing this text and translation.

Glossary

(Skt = Sanskrit; Tib = Tibetan)

Akshobhya (*Skt; Tib: Mi-kyö-pa,* "Imperturbable"). One of the five *dhyani* buddhas, or heads of the five buddha families, who represent the fully purified *skandhas,* or aggregates, of form, feeling, recognition, compositional factors, and consciousness. Akshobhya is blue in color, represents the fully purified aggregate of consciousness, and is lord of the vajra family.

Ajatashatru (*Skt*). Early Indian king who imprisoned and killed his father, Bimbisara. Realizing the enormity of this sin and guided by the Buddha, he purified this negativity and became an arhat.

Angulimala (*Skt*). A character in a classic Dharma story of choosing the wrong guru and committing horrendous actions. In this case, he killed 999 people and made a rosary out of their thumbs. He was prevented by the Buddha from killing his thousandth victim, which, according to the wrong guru, would have led him to liberation. He was able to purify and become an arhat.

arhat (*Skt*). Literally, "foe destroyer." A person who has destroyed his or her delusions and attained liberation from cyclic existence.

Avalokiteshvara (*Skt; Tib: Chenrezig*). The buddha of compassion. A male meditational deity embodying fully enlightened compassion.

bodhicitta (*Skt*). The altruistic determination to reach enlightenment for the sole purpose of enlightening all sentient beings.

bodhisattva (*Skt*). Someone whose spiritual practice is directed toward the achievement of enlightenment. One who possesses the compassionate motivation of *bodhicitta.*

buddha (*Skt*). A fully enlightened being. One who has removed all obscurations veiling the mind and has developed all good qualities to perfection. The first of the Three Jewels of *refuge.* See also *enlightenment.*

central channel. See *shushuma.*

chakra (*Skt*). Energy wheel. A focal point of energy along the central channel (*shushuma*) upon which one's concentration is directed, especially during the completion stage of *highest yoga tantra.* The main chakras are the crown, throat, heart, navel, and secret.

channels (*Skt: nadi*). A constituent of the *vajra* body through which energy winds and drops flow. The central, right, and left are the major channels, which total 72,000 in all.

chu-len (*Tib*). Literally, "taking the essence." Chu-len pills are made of essential ingredients; taking but a few each day, accomplished meditators can remain secluded in retreat for months or years without having to depend upon normal food. See also note 5.

compassion (*Skt: karuna*). The wish for all beings to be separated from their mental and physical suffering. A prerequisite for the development of *bodhicitta.* Compassion is symbolized by the meditational deity *Avalokiteshvara.*

completion stage (*Tib: dzok-rim*). The second of the two stages of *highest yoga tantra,* during which control is gained over the *vajra* body through such practices as inner fire.

daka (*Skt; Tib: kha-dro*). Literally, a "sky-goer." A male being who helps arouse blissful energy in a qualified tantric practitioner.

dakini (*Skt; Tib: kha-dro-ma*). Literally, a "female sky-goer." A female being who helps arouse blissful energy in a qualified tantric practitioner.

damaru (*Skt*). A small hand drum used in tantric practice.

delusion. (*Skt: klesha; Tib: nyön-mong*). An obscuration covering the essentially pure nature of the mind, being thereby responsible for suffering and dissatisfaction; the main delusion is ignorance, out of which grow desirous attachment, hatred, jealousy, and all the other delusions.

Dharma (*Skt*). Spiritual teachings, particularly those of the Buddha. Literally, that which holds one back from suffering. The second of the Three Jewels of *refuge.*

dharmakaya (*Skt*). The "truth body." The mind of a fully enlightened being, which, free of all coverings, remains meditatively absorbed in the direct perception of *emptiness* while simultaneously cognizing all phenomena. One of the three bodies of a *buddha* (see also *nirmanakaya* and *sambhogakaya*).

divine pride. The strong conviction that one has achieved the state of a particular meditational deity. Cf. *generation stage.*

dorje (*Tib; Skt: vajra*). The magical weapon of the Vedic god Indra, made of metal and very sharp and hard; adamantine. A thunderbolt. A tantric implement symbolizing method (compassion or bliss), held in the right hand (the male side), usually in conjunction with a bell, which symbolizes wisdom and is held in the left hand (the female side).

Dorje Khadro (*Tib; Skt: Vajradaka*). A deity who functions to purify negativities through his specific fire puja (*jin-sek*). See also *ngön-dro.*

drops. A constituent of the *vajra* body used in the generation of great bliss. Of the two types, at conception, the red drops are received fromone's mother and the white drops from one's father.

dualistic view. The ignorant view characteristic of the unenlightened mind in which all things are falsely conceived to have concrete self-existence. To such a view, the appearance of an object is mixed with the false image of its being independent or self-existent, thereby leading to further dualistic views concerning subject and object, self and other, this and that, etc.

dzok-rim (*Tib*). See *completion stage.*

ego-grasping. The ignorant compulsion to regard one's self, or I, as permanent, self-existent, and independent of all other phenomena.

empowerment. See *initiation.*

emptiness. See *sunyata.*

enlightenment (*Skt: bodhi*). Full awakening; buddhahood. The ultimate goal of Buddhist practice, attained when all limitations have been removed from the mind and all one's positive potential has been realized. It is a state characterized by unlimited compassion, skill, and wisdom.

four classes of tantra. The division of tantra into *kriya* (action), *carya* (performance), *yoga,* and *anuttara yoga* (highest yoga).

Geluk (*Tib*). The Virtuous Order. The order of Tibetan Buddhism founded by Lama *Tsong Khapa* and his disciples in the early fifteenth century.

generation stage (*Tib: kye-rim*). The first of the two stages of *highest yoga tantra,* during which one cultivates the clear appearance and divine pride of one's chosen meditational deity.

graduated path (*Tib: lam-rim*). A presentation of *Shakyamuni Buddha's* teachings in a form suitable for the step-by-step training of a disciple. The lam-rim was first formulated by the great Indian teacher Atisha (Dipankara Shrijnana, 982–1055) when he came to Tibet in 1042.

guru (*Skt; Tib: lama*). A spiritual guide or teacher. One who shows a disciple the path to *liberation* and *enlightenment.* In *tantra,* one's teacher is seen as inseparable from the meditational deity and the Three Jewels of *refuge.* See also *root guru.*

guru yoga (*Skt*). The fundamental tantric practice, whereby one's *guru* is seen as identical with the *buddhas,* one's personal meditational deity, and the essential nature of one's own mind.

Heruka Chakrasamvara (*Skt; Tib: Kor-lo Dem-chog*). Male meditational deity from the mother tantra class of *highest yoga tantra.* He is the principal deity connected with the Heruka Vajrasattva practice and was Lama Yeshe's *yi-dam.*

highest yoga tantra (*Skt: anuttara-yoga tantra*). The fourth and supreme division of tantric practice, consisting of the *generation* and *completion stages.* Through this practice, one can attain full *enlightenment* within one lifetime.

Hinayana (*Skt*). Literally, the "Small Vehicle." It is one of the two general divisions of Buddhism. Hinayana practitioners' motivation for following the *Dharma* path is principally their intense wish for personal liberation from conditioned existence, or *samsara.* Cf. *Mahayana.*

initiation. Transmission received from a tantric master allowing a disciple to engage in the practices of a particular meditational deity. It is also referred to as an empowerment.

inner fire. (*Tib: tum-mo*). The energy residing at the navel *chakra,* aroused during the *completion stage* of *highest yoga tantra* and used to bring the energy winds into the *central channel.* It is also called inner or psychic heat.

inner offering (*Tib: nang-chö*). A tantric offering whose basis of transformation is one's five aggregates visualized as the five meats and the five nectars. While the relevant inner offering *mantra* of the particular deity is recited (e.g., in Heruka-associated practices it is OM KHANDA ROHI HUM HUM PHAT), the basis is purified, transformed, and magnified by *mantra, mudra,* and concentration. The external support for this meditation is often a blessed inner offering pill (*nang-chö ril-bu*) dissolved in black tea or alcohol.

insight meditation (*Pali: vipassana*). The principal meditation taught in the *Thervada* tradition and is based on the Buddha's teachings on the four foundations of mindfulness. It is sometimes called mindfulness meditation. In the *Mahayana*, *Vipasyana* (*Skt*) has a different connotation, where it means investigation of and familiarization with the actual way in which things exist and is used to develop the wisdom of *emptiness*.

jor-chö (*Tib*). The preparatory rites (see *Liberation in the Palm of Your Hand*, pp. 131–247, and Sopa, Geshe Lhundup, and Hopkins, Jeffrey. *Cutting Through Appearances*. Ithaca: Snow Lion, 1989).

Kagyu (*Tib*). The order of Tibetan Buddhism founded in the eleventh century by *Marpa*, *Milarepa*, Gampopa, and their followers.

kapala (*Skt; Tib: tö-pa*). Skull cup, e.g., the one held by Yum Dorje Nyem-ma.

karma (*Skt; Tib: lä*). Action; the working of cause and effect, whereby positive actions produce happiness and negative actions produce suffering.

kriya (*Skt*). First of the *four classes of tantra;* action tantra.

kundalini (*Skt*). Blissful energy dormant within the physical body, aroused through tantric practice and used to generate penetrative insight into the true nature of reality.

kusha (*Skt*). Kind of long-stranded grass used under the retreat seat, during tantric *initiations*, and for making brooms in India. *Shakyamuni Buddha* made a seat out of kusha grass when he meditated under the *bodhi* tree at Bodhgaya and attained enlightenment.

kye-rim (*Tib*). See *generation stage*.

lama (*Tib*). See *guru*.

lam-rim (*Tib*). See *graduated path*.

liberation. See *nirvana*.

Madhyamaka (*Skt*). The *middle way*; a system of analysis founded by *Nagarjuna*, based on the *prajñaparamita sutras* of *Shakyamuni Buddha*, and considered to be the supreme presentation of the wisdom of emptiness.

Manjushri (*Skt; Tib: Jam-pel-yang*). Male meditational deity embodying fully enlightened wisdom.

maha-anuttara (*Skt*). Also called *anuttara*. See *four classes of tantra* and *highest yoga tantra*. It is divided into *generation* and *completion stages*.

Mahayana (*Skt*). Literally, the "Great Vehicle." It is one of the two general divisions of Buddhism. Mahayana practitioners' motivation for following the *Dharma* path is principally their intense wish for all mother *sentient beings* to be liberated from conditioned existence, or *samsara,* and to attain the full *enlightenment* of buddhahood. The Mahayana has two divisions: *Paramitayana,* or *Sutrayana,* and *Vajrayana.* Cf. *Hinayana.*

mahamudra (*Skt; Tib: chag-chen*). The great seal. A profound system of meditation upon the mind and the ultimate nature of reality.

mandala (*Skt; Tib: khyil-khor*). A circular diagram symbolic of the entire universe. The abode of a meditational deity.

mantra (*Skt*). Literally, protection of the mind. Mantras are Sanskrit syllables recited in conjunction with the practice of a particular meditational deity that embody the qualities of that deity.

mantra rosary. A *mantra* visualized as a rosary, its syllables representing beads; usually circular, as in the syllables of the one hundred syllable mantra standing around the edge of the moon disc.

Marpa (*Tib;* 1012–96). Founder of the *Kagyu* tradition of Tibetan Buddhism. He was a renowned tantric master and translator, and a disciple of Naropa and the *guru* of Milarepa.

middle way. The view presented in *Shakyamuni Buddha's prajñaparamita sutras* and elucidated by *Nagarjuna* that all phenomena are dependent arisings, thereby avoiding the mistaken extremes of self-existence and non-existence, or eternalism and nihilism. Cf. *Madhyamaka.*

Milarepa (*Tib;* 1040–1123). Foremost disciple of *Marpa,* famous for his intense practice, devotion to his *guru,* attainment of *enlightenment* in his lifetime, and his many songs of spiritual realization.

mudra (*Skt; Tib: chag-gya*). Literally, seal, token. A symbolic hand gesture, endowed with power not unlike a *mantra.* A tantric consort.

Nagarjuna (*Skt*). The second century AD Indian Buddhist philosopher who propounded the *Madhyamaka* philosophy of *emptiness.*

nang-chö (*Tib*). See *inner offering.*

ngön-dro (*Tib*). Preliminary practice(s) found in all schools of Tibetan Buddhism, usually done 100,000 times each; the four main ones are recitation of the *refuge* formula, *mandala* offerings, prostrations, and Vajrasattva *mantra* recitation. The

Geluk tradition adds five more: *guru* yoga, water bowl offerings, Damtsig Dorje purifying meditation, making *tsa-tsas* (small sacred images, usually made of clay), and the *Dorje Khadro* burnt offering (*jin-sek*).

nirmanakaya (*Skt*). The "emanation body"; the form in which the enlightened mind appears in order to benefit ordinary beings. One of the three bodies of a *buddha.* See also *dharmakaya* and *sambhogakaya.*

nirvana (*Skt; Tib: thar-pa*). The state of complete *liberation* from *samsara*; the goal of a practitioner seeking his or her own freedom from suffering (see *Hinayana*). "Lower nirvana" is used to refer to this state of self-liberation, while "higher nirvana" refers to the supreme attainment of the full *enlightenment* of buddhahood.

Nyingma (*Tib*). The "ancient" order of Tibetan Buddhism, which traces its teachings back to the time of Padma Sambhava, the eighth century AD Indian tantric master invited to Tibet by King Trisong Detsen to clear away the influences obstructing the establishment of Buddhism. This school includes in its canon works and translations dating from the early period of the dissemination of Buddhism in Tibet.

pandit (*Skt*). Scholar; learned man.

Paramitayana (*Skt*). The "Perfection Vehicle"; one of the two division of the *Mahayana.* This is the gradual path to *enlightenment* traversed by *bodhisattvas* practicing the six perfections of charity, morality, patience, effort, concentration, and wisdom, through the ten bodhisattva levels (*bhumis*) over countless eons of rebirths in *samsara* for the benefit of all *sentient beings.* It is also called *Sutrayana.* See also *Vajrayana.*

prajñaparamita (*Skt*). The "perfection of wisdom"; the *p. sutras* are the teachings of *Shakyamuni Buddha* in which the wisdom of *emptiness* and the path of the *bodhisattva* are set forth. The basis of *Nagarjuna's* philosophy.

pratimoksha (*Skt*). See *vows.*

puja (*Skt*). Literally, "offering." The word is often used loosely, as in "Let's do a puja," to refer to performing a ritual, such as the *Guru Puja* (*Offering to the Spiritual Master; Tib: Lama Chöpa*), or reciting a *sadhana,* such as the *Heruka Vajrasattva* sadhana in this book.

refuge. The door to the *Dharma* path. A Buddhist takes refuge in the Three Jewels of *Buddha, Dharma,* and *Sangha,* fearing the sufferings of *samsara* and believing that the Three Jewels have the power to lead him or her out of suffering, to happiness, *liberation,* or *enlightenment.*

root guru (*Tib: tsa-wäi lama*). The teacher who has had the greatest influence upon a particular disciple's entering or following the spiritual path.

sadhana (*Skt*). method of accomplishment; the step-by-step instructions for practicing the meditations related to a particular meditational deity.

samadhi (*Skt*). See *single-pointed concentration.*

samaya (*Skt; Tib: dam-tsig*). Sacred word of honor; the pledges and commitments made by a disciple at an initiation to keep tantric vows for life or to perform certain practices connected with the deity, such as daily sadhana recitation, or offering the *Guru Puja* on the tenth and the twenty-fifth of each Tibetan month.

sambhogakaya (*Skt*). The "enjoyment body"; the form in which the enlightened mind appears in order to benefit highly realized *bodhisattvas.* One of the three bodies of a *buddha.* See also *dharmakaya* and *nirmanakaya.*

samsara (*Skt; Tib: khor-wa*). Cyclic existence; the six realms of conditioned existence, three lower—hell, hungry spirit (*Skt: preta*), and animal—and three upper—human, demi-god, and god. It is the beginningless, recurring cycle of death and rebirth under the control of *delusion* and *karma* and fraught with suffering. It also refers to the contaminated aggregates of a *sentient being.*

Sangha (*Skt*). Spiritual community; the third of the Three Jewels of *refuge.* Absolute Sangha are those who have directly realized *emptiness;* relative Sangha are ordained monks and nuns.

secret mantra (*Tib: sang-ngak*). See *tantra.*

seed syllable. In tantric visualizations, a Sanskrit syllable arising out of *emptiness* and out of which the meditational deity in turn arises. A single syllable representing a deity's entire *mantra.*

sentient being. Any unenlightened being; any being whose mind is not completely free from gross and subtle ignorance.

Shakyamuni Buddha (563–483 B.C.). Fourth of the one thousand founding buddhas of this present world age. Born a prince of the Shakya clan in North India, he taught the *sutra* and *tantra* paths to *liberation* and full *enlightenment;* founder of what came to be known as Buddhism. (From the *Skt: buddha*—"fully awake.")

shi-dak (*Tib*). Landlord; place owner. Buddhism teaches that each place has associated with it a *sentient being* who considers that he owns it. Offerings are made to this being to request the temporary use of that place for, e.g., retreat.

shushuma (or *avadhuti, Skt; Tib: tsa uma*). The *central channel*, or *nadi*, which runs from the crown of the head to the secret chakra. It is the major energy channel of the *vajra* body, visualized as a hollow tube of light in front of the spine (see chapter 3).

single-pointed concentration (*Skt: samadhi*). A state of deep meditative absorption; single-pointed concentration on the actual nature of things, free from discursive thought and dualistic conceptions.

sunyata (*Skt*). The absence of all false ideas about how things exist; specifically, the lack of the apparent independent, self-existence of phenomena. Usually translated as *emptiness* or voidness.

sutra (*Skt*). A discourse of *Shakyamuni Buddha;* the pre-tantric division of Buddhist teachings stressing the cultivation of *bodhicitta* and the practice of the six perfections. See also *Paramitayana.*

tantra (*Skt; Tib: gyüd*). Literally, thread, or continuity. The texts of the *secret mantra* teachings of Buddhism; often used to refer to these teachings themselves. Cf. *Vajrayana.*

tathagata (*Skt; Tib: de-zhin shek-pa*). Literally, one who has realized suchness; a *buddha.*

Theravada (*Skt*). One of the eighteen schools into which the *Hinayana* split not long after *Shakyamuni Buddha's* death; the dominant school today, prevalent in Thailand, Sri Lanka, and Burma, and well represented in the West.

torma (*Tib*). An offering cake used in tantric rituals. In Tibet, tormas were usually made of *tsampa*, but other edibles such as biscuits and so forth will suffice.

tsampa (*Tib*). Roasted barley flour; a Tibetan staple food.

tsok (*Tib*). Literally, gathering—a gathering of offering substances and a gathering of disciples to make the offering.

Tsong Khapa, Lama Je (1357–1417). Founder of the *Geluk* tradition of Tibetan Buddhism, and revitalizer of many *sutra* and *tantra* lineages and the monastic tradition in Tibet.

tum-mo (*Tib*). See *inner fire.*

Vajradhara (*Skt; Tib: Dorje Chang*). Male meditational deity; the form through which *Shakyamuni Buddha* revealed the teachings of *secret mantra.*

Vajrasattva (*Skt; Tib: Dorje Sem-pa*). Male meditational deity symbolizing the inherent purity of all *buddhas.* A major tantric purification practice for removing obstacles created by negative *karma* and the breaking of *vows.*

Vajravarahi (*Skt; Tib: Dorje Phag-mo*). Female meditational deity; consort of *Heruka.*

Vajrayana (*Skt*). The adamantine vehicle; the second of the two *Mahayana* paths. It is also called *Tantrayana* or *Mantrayana.* This is the quickest vehicle of Buddhism, as it allows practitioners to attain *enlightenment* within one lifetime. See also *tantra*

Vinaya (*Skt; Tib: dül-wa*). The division of the Buddhist scriptures concerned with monastic discipline—the rules for the behavior of monks and nuns and the conduct of their communal business.

Vipassana (*Pali*). See *insight meditation.*

vows. Precepts taken on the basis of *refuge* at all levels of Buddhist practice. *Pratimoksha* precepts (vows of individual liberation) are the main vows in the *Hinayana* tradition and are taken by monks, nuns, and lay people; they are the basis of all other vows. *Bodhisattva* and tantric precepts are the main vows in the *Mahayana* tradition. See also *Vinaya.*

Yamantaka (*Skt;* also *Vajra Bhairava; Tib: Dorje Jig-je*). Male meditaional deity from the father tantra class of *highest yoga tantra.*

yana (*Skt*). Literally, vehicle; a spiritual path that takes you from where you are to where you want to be. See also *Hinayana, Mahayana,* etc.

yi-dam (T*ib*). Literally, "mind-bound." One's own personal, main—or, as Lama Yeshe used to say, favorite—deity for tantric practice. The deity with which you have the strongest connection.

CHRONOLOGY

INTELLECTUALS, BEWARE!

This "word of caution to the intellectual" was written by Lama in 1974, as the preface to a short Chenrezig sadhana he had composed during his and Lama Zopa Rinpoche's first visit to Australia, and augmented in 1976 for use with the Heruka Vajrasattva sadhana.

Parts 1& 2

A Commentary to the Heruka Vajrasattva Sadhana and Retreat Instructions, April-May 1974, Kopan Monastery, Nepal. Archive number 000048.

Additional Retreat Instructions (from Chenrezig Retreat Instructions), probably 1976, Chenrezig Institute, Australia. Archive number 000730.

Part 3

1. Combination of Vajrasattva Explanation, 6 February 1974, and Vajrasattva Guru Yoga, 28 January 1976, both Kopan Monastery. Archive numbers 000173 and 000051 respectively.

2. Vajrasattva Initiation, June, 1977, Chenrezig Institute. Archive number 000805.

3. Vajrasattva Commentary, July 1980, Vajrapani Institute, USA. Archive number 000620.

4. Vajrasattva Explanation during Vajrayogini Commentary, excerpt, 2 April 1983, Tushita Retreat Centre, India. Archive number 000320.

5. Introduction to Vajrasattva Initiation, 20 April 1983, Tushita Retreat Centre. Archive number 000964.

6. Introduction to Vajrasattva Initiation, 17 July 1983, Vajrapani Institute. Archive number 000071.

Part 4

Ritual text composed 19 January 1982, Bodhgaya, India.

Commentary and Oral Transmission of the Heruka Vajrasattva Tsok, 2

February 1982, Bodhgaya. Archive number 000175.

A Brief Explanation of Tsok, 22 April 1983, Tushita Retreat Centre. Archive number 000965.

Commentary on the Heruka Vajrasattva Tsok, 3 to 31 July 1983, Vajrapani Institute. Archive number 000179.

PHOTOGRAPHS OF LAMA YESHE

Frontispiece	Vajrapani Institute, USA, 1983
Page 2	Vajrapani Institute, USA, 1983
Page 68	India, ca. 1970
Page 100	Melbourne, Australia, 1974
Page 158	(with Lama Zopa Rinpoche), Solu Khumbu, Nepal, 1971

Suggested Further Reading

Books by Lama Yeshe

The Bliss of Inner Fire. Edited by Robina Courtin and Ailsa Cameron. Boston: Wisdom Publications, 1995.

Introduction to Tantra: A Vision of Totality. Compiled and edited by Jonathan Landaw. Boston: Wisdom Publications, 1987.

Silent Mind, Holy Mind (revised edition). Edited by Jonathan Landaw. Boston: Wisdom Publications, (1979) 1995.

——— and Zopa Rinpoche. *Wisdom Energy.* Edited by Jonathan Landaw and Alexander Berzin. Boston: Wisdom Publications, (1976) 1982.

——— et al. *Wisdom Energy 2.* Boston: Wisdom Publications, 1979.

Transcripts by Lama Yeshe

Gyalwa Gyatso. Boston: Wisdom Publications, (1983) 1984.

Life, Death and After Death. Boston: Wisdom Publications, (1984) 1990.

Light of Dharma. Boston: Wisdom Publications, (1984) 1993.

Transference of Consciousness at the Time of Death. Boston: Wisdom Publications, (1985) 1991.

About Lama Yeshe

Reincarnation: The Boy Lama. Vicki Mackenzie. London: Bloomsbury, 1988.

The Kindness of the Guru. Lama Zopa Rinpoche. Transcript. Boston: Wisdom Publications, (1984) 1993.

GENERAL BUDDHISM

Gyatso, Tenzin, the Fourteenth Dalai Lama. *Kindness, Clarity, and Insight.* Translated and edited by Jeffrey Hopkins. Ithaca: Snow Lion Publications, 1984.

———. *The World of Tibetan Buddhism.* Translated, edited, and annotated by Geshe Thupten Jinpa. Boston: Wisdom Publications, 1995.

Hopkins, Jeffrey. *The Tantric Distinction.* Boston: Wisdom Publications, 1984.

McDonald, Kathleen. *How to Meditate.* Edited by Robina Courtin. Boston: Wisdom Publications, 1984.

Pabongka Rinpoche. *Liberation in the Palm of Your Hand.* Edited in the Tibetan by Trijang Rinpoche. Translated by Michael Richards. Boston: Wisdom Publications, 1991.

Wallace, B. Alan. *Tibetan Buddhism From the Ground Up.* Boston: Wisdom Publications, 1993.

Wangyel, Geshe. *The Door of Liberation.* Boston: Wisdom Publications, 1995.

Zopa Rinpoche, Lama. *The Direct and Unmistaken Method.* Boston: Wisdom Publications, 1990.

———. *The Door to Satisfaction.* Edited by Ailsa Cameron and Robina Courtin. Boston: Wisdom Publications, 1994.

———. *Transforming Problems into Happiness.* Edited by Ailsa Cameron and Robina Courtin. Boston: Wisdom Publications, 1993.

TANTRIC BUDDHISM

Cozort, Daniel. *Highest Yoga Tantra.* Ithaca: Snow Lion Publications, 1986.

Tsong-ka-pa, Tenzin Gyatso, and Jeffrey Hopkins. *Tantra in Tibet: The Great Exposition of Secret Mantra—Volume 1.* Ithaca: Snow Lion Publications, (1977) 1987.

———. *Deity Yoga in Action and Performance Tantra.* Ithaca: Snow Lion Publications, (1981, as *The Yoga of Tibet*), 1987.

Wisdom Publications

Wisdom Publications is a non-profit publisher of books on Buddhism, Tibet, and related East-West themes. Our titles are published in appreciation of Buddhism as a living philosophy and with the special commitment to preserve and transmit important works from all the major Buddhist traditions.

If you would like more information or a copy of our mail order catalogue, and to be kept informed about future publications, please write to us at: 361 Newbury Street, Boston, Massachusetts, 02115, USA.

The Wisdom Trust

As a non-profit publisher, Wisdom is dedicated to the publication of fine Dharma books for the benefit of all sentient beings. We depend upon sponsors in order to publish books like the one you are holding in your hand.

If you would like to make a donation to the Wisdom Trust Fund to help us continue our Dharma work or to receive information about opportunities for planned giving, please write to our Boston office.

Thank you so much.

Wisdom is a non-profit, charitable 501(c)(3) organization and a part of the Foundation for the Preservation of the Mahayana Tradition (FPMT).

THE LAMA YESHE PUBLISHING FUND

LAMA THUBTEN YESHE (1935–84) was the founder of Wisdom Publications and the Foundation for the Preservation of the Mahayana Tradition (FPMT). Over the course of his fifteen-year contact with Western students of Buddhism he gave hundreds of teachings: general talks, discourses on the graduated path to enlightenment, sutra teachings, and especially tantric commentaries. All these teachings have been taped and transcribed and currently reside on the computers of the Wisdom Archive.

WISDOM PUBLICATIONS, a 501(c)(3) tax-deductible, non-profit organization, has established the LAMA YESHE PUBLISHING FUND to publish the teachings of Lama Yeshe in the form of books, such as *The Tantric Path of Purification, Silent Mind Holy Mind, Wisdom Energy, Introduction to Tantra,* and *The Bliss of Inner Fire.* This fund will also allow Wisdom to publish in book form the thousands of Archive pages of teachings of Lama Thubten Zopa Rinpoche—Lama Yeshe's heart disciple and spiritual head of the FPMT—books such as *Transforming Problems* and *The Door to Satisfaction.*

If you would like to make a contribution of any kind to the Lama Yeshe Publishing Fund, please contact Wisdom at 361 Newbury Street, Boston, MA 02115, USA; telephone (617) 536-3358; fax (617) 536-1897. Thank you so much for your support.

Wisdom is making available a six-hour video series of Lama Yeshe's 1983 Heruka Vajrasattva Tsok commentary at the Vajrapani Institute. If you would like to receive more information about this, please write or call Wisdom Publications.

The Foundation for the Preservation of the Mahayana Tradition

The Foundation for the Preservation of the Mahayana Tradition (FPMT) is an international network of Buddhist centers and activities dedicated to the transmission of Mahayana Buddhism as a practiced and living tradition. The FPMT was founded in 1975 by Lama Thubten Yeshe and Lama Thubten Zopa Rinpoche. It is composed of monasteries, retreat centers, communities, publishing houses, and healing centers, all functioning as a means to benefit others. Teachings, such as those presented in this book, are given at many of these centers.

To receive a complete listing of these centers as well as news about the activities throughout this global network, please request a complimentary copy of the Mandala journal from:

FPMT Central Office
P.O. Box 1778
Soquel, California 95073

Telephone: (408) 476-8435
Fax: (408) 476-4823.

Care of Dharma Books

Dharma books contain the teachings of the Buddha; they have the power to protect against lower rebirth and to point the way to liberation. Therefore, they should be treated with respect—kept off the floor and places where people sit or walk—and not stepped over. They should be covered or protected for transporting and kept in a high, clean place separate from more "mundane" materials. Other objects should not be placed on top of Dharma books and materials. Licking the fingers to turn pages is considered bad form (and negative karma). If it is necessary to dispose of Dharma materials, they should be burned rather than thrown in the trash. When burning Dharma texts, it is considered skillful to first recite a prayer or mantra, such as OM, AH, HUNG. Then, you can visualize the letters of the texts (to be burned) absorbing into the AH, and the AH absorbing into you. After that, you can burn the texts.

These considerations may also be kept in mind for Dharma artwork, as well as the written teachings and artwork of other religions.

Wisdom Publications